D1516740

Progress in Neurotherapeutics and Neuropsychopharmacology

Published annually, volumes in this series provide readers with updates of recent clinical trial results, impacts of trials on guidelines and evidence-based practice, advances in trial methodologies, and the evolution of biomarkers in trials. The series focuses on trials in neurotherapeutics, including disease-modifying and symptomatic agents for neurological diseases, psychopharmacological management of neurological and psychiatric illnesses, and non-drug treatments. Each article is authored by a leader in the area of neurotherapeutics and clinical trials, and the series is guided by an Editor-in-Chief and Editorial Board with broad experience in drug development and neuropsychopharmacology. *Progress in Neurotherapeutics and Neuropsychopharmacology* is an essential update of recent trials in all aspects of the management of neurological and neuropsychiatric disorders, and will be an invaluable resource for practising neurologists as well as clinical and translational neuroscientists. Articles also available at http: www.cambridge.org/jid_PNN

Editor-in-Chief

Jeffrey L. Cummings, MD
Department of Neurology and Psychiatry and Biobehavioral Sciences,
David Geffen School of Medicine at UCLA,
Los Angeles, CA, USA

Editorial Board

Peter Goadsby, MD, PhD

Institute of Neurology, National Hospital for Neurology and Neurosurgery, London, UK

Karl Kieburtz, MD, FAAN

Department of Neurology, University of Rochester Medical Center, Rochester, NY, USA

Joseph Masdeu, MD, PhD, FAAN

Department of Neurology, University of Navarre Medical School Pamplona, Spain

Gary Tollefson, MD, PhD

Orexigen Therapeutics, Inc. and Department of Psychiatry, Indiana University School of Medicine, Indianapolis, IN, USA

Progress in Neurotherapeutics and Neuropsychopharmacology

VOL. 1   2006

Editor-in-Chief

Jeffrey L. Cummings, MD

Department of Neurology and Biobehavioral Sciences,

David Geffen School of Medicine at UCLA,

Los Angeles, CA, USA

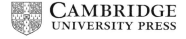

PUBLISHED BY THE PRESS SYNDICATE OF THE UNIVERSITY OF CAMBRIDGE
The Pitt Building, Trumpington Street, Cambridge, United Kingdom

CAMBRIDGE UNIVERSITY PRESS
The Edinburgh Building, Cambridge CB2 2RU, UK
40 West 20th Street, New York, NY 10011-4211, USA
477 Williamstown Road, Port Melbourne, VIC 3207, Australia
Ruiz de Alarcón 13, 28014 Madrid, Spain
Dock House, The Waterfront, Cape Town 8001, South Africa

http://www.cambridge.org

© Cambridge University Press 2006

First published 2006

Printed in the United Kingdom at the University Press, Cambridge

A catalogue record for this book is available from the British Library

ISBN 9780521862530 (0521862531)
ISSN 17482321

Every effort has been made in preparing this book to provide accurate and
up-to-date information which is in accord with accepted standards and
practice at the time of publication. Nevertheless, the authors, editors
and publisher can make no warranties that the information contained
herein is totally free from error, not least because clinical standards are
constantly changing through research and regulation. The authors, editors
and publisher therefore disclaim all liability for direct or consequential
damages resulting from the use of material contained in this book. Readers
are strongly advised to pay careful attention to information provided by
the manufacturer of any drugs or equipment that they plan to use.

Acknowledgments

I would like to acknowledge the assistance of the editorial board in guiding the concepts and developing the content of *Progress in Neurotherapeutics and Neuropsychopharmacology* (PNN). Each member of the editorial board brings special expertise to a complex enterprise such as PNN. I gratefully acknowledge the assistance of Karl Kieburtz, Garry Tollefson, Joseph Masdeu, and Peter Goadsby.

I would like to acknowledge Richard Barling and Gavin Swanson at Cambridge University Press for their assistance for reviewing, organizing, and assisting in the development of PNN. Their novel concepts in combining print and electronic publication were particularly helpful in creating this unique approach to publication.

Maria Barceló and Josie Sanchez were of great assistance in organizing the administrative aspects of this volume.

The duties of an editor-in-chief cannot be accomplished without enthusiastic family support. I would like to acknowledge Kate (Xue) Zhong for the love and support that she has brought to my life.

Jeffrey L. Cummings

Kate (Xue) Zhong
For all you are, for all you do

Contents

Progress in Neurotherapeutics and Neuropsychopharmacology, 1:1, ix–xi © 2006 Cambridge University Press
DOI: 10.1017/S1748232105000017   Printed in the United Kingdom

Preface

Progress in Neurotherapeutics and Neuropsychopharmacology (PNN) represents a new concept in content and in publishing. From a publishing point of view, PNN is a unique combination of print and electronic processing to maximize availability of information. Chapters are solicited continuously and placed online after editing. Online, these chapters are in the complete published and citable format. Annually, chapters are collected into a single volume and published in book form. The chapters are available on the shelf or electronically according to the reader's preference. Moreover, there is minimal delay in conveying the information from the author to the reader. The growing archive of on-line chapters will allow readers to review all of the recent information available for specific diseases, biomarkers, or methodologies.

From the content point of view, PNN has a single focus on therapeutic advances through clinical trials. Clinical trials provide information for evidence-based medicine to advance care of patients. PNN will emphasize double-blind, randomized, controlled trials that provide the highest quality data to guide clinical practice. Each chapter will focus on a single trial or a few related trials and will include an interpretation of how the trial results influence contemporary approaches to practice. Articles relevant to advancing trial methodology will be included. Progress in trial design or trial analyses are an important part of the growing literature on clinical trials. In addition, the integration of biomarkers as surrogate outcome measures in clinical trials is a critically important research area, particularly as disease-modifying agents enter the clinical trials arena. PNN will include publications on these methodologic advances. Similarly, improved understanding in the informed consent process, the ethics of clinical trials, and regulatory issues relevant to drug development in clinical trials will be included among PNN contributions.

Alzheimer's disease, Parkinson's disease, multiple sclerosis, epilepsy, migraine, schizophrenia

This first issue of the hard bound edition of PNN includes an exiting array of new trial results. The introductory chapter by the Editor-in-Chief, sets the stage for the progress being made with new therapeutic advances emerging for Alzheimer's disease, Parkinson's disease, multiple sclerosis, epilepsy, migraine, schizophrenia, headache, substance use disorders and many other central nervous system conditions. The phases of drug discovery and development are outlined with Phases II, III, and IV emphasized in PNN covered in greater detail. Contributions in this volume include treatment approaches on neurologic diseases including Parkinson's disease, multiple sclerosis, brain tumors, migraine, amyotrophic lateral sclerosis, and pseudobulbar affect. Idiopathic psychiatric disorders with neuropsychopharmacologic treatments tested in new trials described in the current volume of PNN include schizophrenia and autism.

Discussions of clinical trial methods, development of new treatment approaches, and use of approved medications for new purposes are included in this volume of PNN. Tekin and Lane describe a trial in which rivastigmine – currently approved for treatment of Alzheimer's disease – is used for the treatment of the dementia of Parkinson's disease. Effect sizes may be larger in this condition than in Alzheimer's disease. Stankoff and co-workers investigated the potential utility of modafinil for fatigue in multiple sclerosis and found not benefit using the dose and regimen of this trial. Mason and colleagues present an important trial that contributed to Food and Drug Administration (FDA) approval of temozolomide for treatment of glioblastoma multiforme. Dr. Wiendels and Dr. Ferrari review the evolving types of clinical trials used to assess triptans in acute migraine and note that early treatment is not necessarily the optimal way to conduct a trial. Gordon *et al.* and Jeremy Schefner contribute chapters on minocycline and creatine as potential treatments for amyotrophic lateral sclerosis. Gordon and coworkers provide safety, tolerability, and dosing data critical to construction of a Phase III trial of minocycline. Using a futility type analysis, Schefner showed the effects of creatine were not sufficient to warrant further investigation. This outcome was somewhat surprising given the robust effects of creatine in animal models. Dosing issues will have to be reconsidered before a next step is taken with this agent. Another interesting observation in this trial concerns what patients will choose to do when they are enlisted in a clinical trial that they know is testing a medication that is already available on the market. Urine studies showed that six out of thirty-one patients in the placebo group had creatine levels in their urine suggesting that they had decided to take creatine outside of the context of the trial. Pope contributes an interesting chapter on an experimental agent (AVP-923) consisting of a fixed combination of dextromethorphan and quinidine for the treatment of pseudobulbar affect.

Autism has proven to be treatment resistant but the chapter by Hollander and colleagues suggests that fluoxetine may be beneficial for control of at least some symptom complexes. Several new therapeutic approaches to schizophrenia are included in this volume of PNN. Using a unique clinical trial methodology, Meltzer and colleagues, tested a neurokinin antagonist, a serotonin 2a/2c antagonist, a central cannabinoid antagonist, and a neurotensin antagonist. This strategy allowed optimal use of a common placebo group to facilitate multiple proof-of-concept observations. Negative and cognitive symptoms have become an important focus of treatment research in schizophrenia. Lin and Bodkin (testing selegiline) and Turner and Sahakian (testing modafinil) provide preliminary data that these symptoms complexes may have treatable components. Simpson and coworkers report one of a small number of head-to-head comparisons of atypical antipsychotic agents. Possible earlier onset of effect of ziprasidone and greater cardiovascular morbidity of olanzapine are suggested by this trial.

Several themes emerge from an overview of the clinical trials in this volume of PNN. An exciting observation reported in the study Mason *et al.* is that genetic subtype appeared to have a great effect on treatment responsiveness. This type of information may help to guide treatment choice for individual patients in the future. Another theme concerns disease-modifying agents for treatment of neurodegenerative disorders. Clinical trials of minocycline and creatine in amyotrophic lateral sclerosis (ALS) are reported. The two trials included in the current volume do not show marked benefit but they set the stage for the next step in the development of disease-modifying and neuroprotective therapies. Another emergent theme is the use of symptomatic agents across disease states with common characteristics. Trials using modafanil to treat cognition and attentional shifting in patients with schizophrenia in one trial and to treat fatigue in multiple sclerosis in another are reported. Improvements were seen in schizophrenia but no relief of fatigue was evident on patients with multiple sclerosis. These trials begin to refine our understanding of agents such as modafanil that may have broad application in diseases with cognitive manifestations including the cognitive symptoms of schizophrenia and dementing disorders. Similarly, the use of selegiline as augmentation therapy for antipsychotic medications to treat negative symptoms in patients with schizophrenia is a further example of a medication with uses across multiple neurologic and psychiatric illnesses. Selegiline is used to treat the motor symptoms of Parkinson's disease, to slow the rate of loss of activities of daily living in Alzheimer's disease, and to have antidepressant qualities. The new trial suggests that it may be useful to treat negative symptoms in patients of schizophrenia.

Several barriers to drug development can be identified in the information provided in the clinical trials reviewed in this volume of PNN. Particularly striking is a failure of the ALS mouse model to predict a clinically significant response to creatine in patients with ALS (Jeremy Schefner). Effective drug development strategies will depend on highly predicative animal models and determining the reasons for failures in predictive success can lead to important improvements in drug development.

PNN provides an overview of emerging themes in neurotherapeutics and NPP, and guides insight into treatment advances relevant to the management of patients with a variety of neurologic and psychiatric disorders.

Progress in Neurotherapeutics and Neuropsychopharmacology, 1:1, xii–xiii © 2006 Cambridge University Press
DOI: 10.1017/S1748232105000017   Printed in the United Kingdom

Contributors

Evdokia Anagnostou, MD
Seaver & NY Autism Center of
  Excellence,
Mount Sinai School of Medicine,
NY, USA

William Chaplin, PhD
Seaver & NY Autism Center of
  Excellence,
Mount Sinai School of Medicine,
NY, USA

Michel Clanet
Fédération de Neurologie,
CHU de Toulouse,
France

Jeffrey L. Cummings, MD
University of California,
Los Angeles,
CA, USA

Michel D. Ferrari, MD, PhD
Ledien University Medical Centre,
North Carolina

N.J. Wiendels, MD
Ledien University Medical Centre,
North Carolina

Paul Gordon, MD
Eleanor and Lou Gehrig MDA/ALS
  Research Center,
Columbia, NY, USA

Eric Hollander, MD
Seaver & NY Autism Center of
  Excellence,
Mount Sinai School of Medicine,
NY, USA

Roger Lane
Novartis Pharmaceuticals
  Corporation,
East Hanover,
NJ, USA

Allison Lin, BA
McLean Hospital Harvard Medical
  School,
Boston

Antony Loebel, MD
LAC + USC Medical Center,
Los Angeles,
CA, USA

Catherine Lubetzki
Fédération de Neurologie,
Hopital Pitié-Salpêtrière,
Paris, France

Warren P. Mason, MD
Department of Medicine,
Princess Margaret Hospital, and The
  University of Toronto,
Toronto, Ontario, Canada

Herbert Meltzer, MD
Vanderbilt University School of
  Medicine,
Nashville, TN, USA

Rene O. Mirimanoff, MD
Department of Oncology,
Multidisciplinary Oncology Center,
Centre Hospitalier Universitaire Vaudois,
Lausanne, Switzerland

Roger Stupp, MD
Department of Oncology,
Multidisciplinary Oncology Center,
Centre Hospitalier Universitaire Vaudois,
Lausanne, Switzerland

Robert G. Miller
Eleanor and Lou Gehrig MDA/ALS
  Research Center,
Columbia

Dan H. Moore
Eleanor and Lou Gehrig MDA/ALS
  Research Center,
Columbia

Ann Phillips, PhD
Seaver & NY Autism Center of Excellence,
Mount Sinai School of Medicine,
NY, USA

Laura E. Pope, PhD
Avanir Pharmaceuticals, USA

Barbara J. Sahakian
FmedSci, University of Cambridge,
Cambridge, England

Jeremy Shefner, MD, PhD
SUNY Upstate Medical University,
NY, USA

George Simpson, MD
LAC + USC Medical Center,
Los Angeles, CA, USA

Lewis Warrington MD
LAC + USC Medical Center,
Los Angeles, CA, USA

Bruno Stankoff
Centre d'Investigation Clinique,
Service de Pharmacologie,
Hopital Pitié-Salpêtrière,
Hopital Pitié-Salpêtrière, Paris, France

Roger Stupp, MD
Department of Oncology,
Multidisciplinary Oncology Center,
Centre Hospitalier Universitaire Vaudois,
Lausanne, Switzerland

Erika Swanson, MA
Seaver & NY Autism Center of
  Excellence,
Mount Sinai School of Medicine,
NY, USA

Sibel Tekin, MD
Novartis Pharmaceuticals Corporation,
East Hanover, NJ, USA

Daniel Turner, MD
FmedSci, University of Cambridge,
England

Lewis Warrington MD
LAC + USC Medical Center,
Los Angeles, CA, USA

Stacey Wasserman, MD
Seaver & NY Autism Center of
  Excellence,
Mount Sinai School of Medicine,
NY, USA

N.J. Wiendels, MD
Ledien University Medical Centre,
North Carolina

Ruoyong Yang, MD, PhD
LAC + USC Medical Center,
Los Angeles, CA, USA

Progress in Neurotherapeutics and Neuropsychopharmacology, 1:1, 1–11 © 2006 Cambridge University Press
DOI: 10.1017/S1748232105000029   Printed in the United Kingdom

Introduction to Neurotherapeutics and Neuropsychopharmacology

Jeffrey L. Cummings

Department of Neurology and Psychiatry & Biobehavioral Sciences, Davids Geffen School of Medicine at UCLA, Los Angeles, CA, USA; Email:jcummings@mednet.ucla.edu

Key words: Neurotherapeutics; psychotropics; clinical trials; drug development; Phase II, Phase III.

Introduction

In recent years there has been tremendous progress in advancing new treatments for neurologic and psychiatric illnesses. New agents have emerged for the treatment of Alzheimer's disease, Parkinson's disease, multiple sclerosis, epilepsy, migraine, schizophrenia, bipolar illness, depression, and substance abuse disorders. Advances in understanding of basic pathophysiology and molecular biology of brain disorders have led to increasingly sophisticated target identification that guides drug development. Advances in the basic neuroscience and disease mechanisms have been particularly obvious in the neurologic disorders where there is an ever improving understanding of the underlying mechanisms of brain function and brain disease.

Progress in neurotherapeutics has occurred in concert with progress in basic science methodologies, neuroimaging, clinical trial design, and trial analysis. There is an increasing enthusiasm for clinical trials that provide highly credible data with which to guide evidence-based medicine. The United States Food and Drug Administration (US FDA) requires a close link between the clinical trial population tested and the specific indication for which the agent will be approved. This contributes to the proliferation of clinical trials, as industry sponsors of trials seek to expand the populations for which their products are indicated. An increasing number of patients and physicians are involved in clinical trials. Advancing clinical trial methodology has itself become a major endeavor.

Correspondence should be addressed to: Jeffrey L. Cummings, MD, Department of Neurology, Reed Neurological Research Center, UCLA, 710 Westwood Plaza, Los Angeles, CA 90095 1769, USA; Email: jcummings@mednet.ucla.edu.

Progress in Neurotherapeutics and Neuropsychopharmacology has two objectives:

1. to provide a continuous update of the clinical trials that can be used to inform and improve the care of patients with neurologic and psychiatric illnesses

2. to provide an update on clinical trial methodologies, designs, and outcome assessments.

This article provides an overview of the themes emerging in current neuropsychopharmacology and the associated clinical trials.

Drug Discovery and Development

The process of drug discovery and development begins with the identification of a human disease or condition, and an unmet need in the form of inadequate treatment (Figure 1). The objective of neurotherapeutic drug discovery and development is to identify new treatments that will improve the quality of life (QOL) of patients suffering from neurologic and psychiatric disorders. Advances in molecular genetics, basic cell biology, brain connectivity, neurologic chemistry, and brain

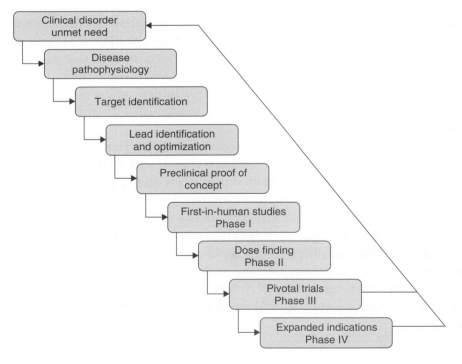

Fig. 1.
Cycle of drug discovery and development.

imaging have continued to an improved understanding of the neurobiologic basis of normal brain function, and of major neurologic disorders.

Characterization of basic disease processes facilitates a focused search for pharmacologically manipulable targets around which a drug development program can be built. Once a neurochemical deficit or alteration in enzymatic activity, transmitter receptor or transporter physiology, gene product abnormality, or protein production or folding disturbance is identified compounds can be sought that ameliorate the consequences of these abnormal mechanisms. For example, the current concepts of Alzheimer's disease suggest that the aggregation of amyloid beta protein in the brain is the principal cause of the disorder. Many current drug development programs are aimed at modifying this process (Cummings, 2004). After a target has been identified and compounds that may potentially modify the basic processes have been found, the "druggability" of these chemical entities must be determined. Factors such as whether they can cross the blood–brain barrier, are likely to have a half-life that will support clinical application, have biochemical features commonly associated with side-effects, or have properties that interfere with establishing clinically useful formulations are reviewed to determine if the chemical entity is plausible as a drug candidate. In some cases the molecular structure of the candidate entity can be modified in the process of lead optimization to produce a compound or a series of compounds that can be advanced in the drug development process.

Candidate compounds can come from a wide variety of sources. Pharmaceutical companies, biotechnology companies, and some federal agencies maintain compound libraries that may be screened for the properties sought to intervene in an identified pathophysiologic process. Modern techniques of high-throughput screening allow thousands or tens of thousands of compounds to be screened rapidly. *In silico* design of new molecular entities using advanced computerized modeling techniques is also advancing. Designer drugs with the desired chemical characteristics can then be produced by medicinal chemists. Herbal medicine and folk treatments, such as Chinese traditional medicine, are another source of compounds. Empirical observations often made over thousands of years have suggested specific activities of compounds to be tested. The variable occurrence of neurologic and psychiatric disorders among world populations may suggest environmental or dietary substances that may be tested for potential pharmaceutical development. Many drugs are developed not through an improved understanding of basic pathophysiologic mechanisms but on the basis of empirical observations of drugs used for one clinical condition and re-purposed for another. For example, the ability of propranolol to reduce essential tremor was discovered when this agent was used in patients with cardiovascular disease who incidentally suffered from a tremor disorder. Another common pathway for drug development is to refine an existing compound to increase efficacy or decrease side-effects. This pathway is particularly common as a mechanism for developing new psychotropic compounds where relatively minor modifications in molecular structure have led to the new antipsychotics, antidepressants, anxiolytics and hypnotics. Finally, biologic agents such as antibodies are increasingly being investigated for their potential utility in treating neuropsychiatric illnesses.

Once lead optimization has occurred, further pre-clinical testing of the chemical entity in laboratory animals is indicated (Figure 1) (Ng, 2004; Lee *et al.*, 2003). Absorption, distribution, metabolism, and excretion (ADME) are investigated to determine the effects of the body on the drug. Toxicologic investigations are also pursued to determine the effect of the drug on the body. Assessments are typically made in at least three species to allow for interspecies variability in drug metabolism and toxicity. Only those agents with pharmacokinetic characteristics suggestive of a compound that can be used successfully in human beings are advanced to the next stage.

Simultaneously with the testing of pharmacokinetic properties, pharmaco-dynamic characteristics are also typically investigated in models of the disease the agent is intended to treat. Effects on prepulse inhibition or learned helplessness assist in predicting antipsychotic and antidepressant qualities, respectively. Lesioning of the nucleus basalis creates a cholinergic deficit and allows testing of compounds for their potential beneficial cholinergic effects in this model. Medical proficiency training program (MPTP) is used to create models for some aspects of parkinsonism. There is increasing enthusiasm for the use of transgenic animals created by the introduction of human mutations into the experimental animal (usually a mouse, but other species also may be used) genome. These animals are fated to develop aspects of the human disease against which the effects of candidate compounds can be tested.

Agents with promising pharmacokinetic and pharmacodynamic profiles are advanced to first-in-human studies in Phase I clinical trials (Figure 1). Normal healthy volunteers are typically used in these trials in an attempt to determine if candidate agents have safety effects or limited tolerability that would make further human testing impractical. Single-dose studies of increasing doses of the drug are typically followed by longer multiple-dose studies. Pharmacokinetic data are collected to determine the half-life, the maximum concentration area under-the-curve, and other parameters. Vital signs, blood and serum measures, electrocardiograms and cognitive functions, are carefully followed to detect any adverse effects. Computerized neuropsychologic assessments and electroencephalography may assist in determining which compounds pass the blood–brain barrier and have either adverse or beneficial central nervous system (CNS) effects. In some cases, Phase I studies called "bridging" studies may be conducted with the intended patient population.

After the completion of Phase I, compounds are advanced to Phase II if they have acceptable tolerability, safety, and pharmacokinetic properties (Ng, 2004; Lee *et al.*, 2003). Phase II studies involve a specific patient population and are intended to garner additional safety and tolerability information in this specific patient group as well as to determine the doses and formulations that will be used in Phase III clinical trials. Phase II studies also generate preliminary efficacy information that may assist in determining whether a compound is advanced to Phase III. Carefully executed Phase II studies are critical since inadequate testing of a variety of doses and optimal formulations may lead to inappropriate abandonment of a compound or choice of sub-optimal doses for Phase III.

Phase III is the final phase of drug development prior to presenting a new chemical entity to the FDA for review and potential approval for marketing (Ng, 2004; Lee *et al.*, 2003) (Figure 1). These trials are "pivotal" trials in which the doses and formulations to be marketing are tested for efficacy. Standardized disease or syndrome definitions, well-established outcomes with valid and reliable instruments, and sophisticated data management and pre-specified data analytic strategies are required for FDA presentation. Drug safety and tolerability are comprehensively assessed.

Once the FDA receives and reviews the documentation, it may choose to approve the compound and will base the language of the package insert that describes the specific indications for the approved drug on the data presented from the Phase III clinical trials. This language is critically important to industry sponsors since marketing can occur only for approved indications of the drug. So-called "off label" use of drugs is common but observations derived from "off label" use cannot be incorporated as part of a drug marketing program. The FDA may also view the submitted data as inadequate and choose not to approve the drug or additional data may be requested.

After marketing, the drug is widely used by physicians to treat many patients including individuals not suffering from the disorder the medication was intended to treat. New side-effects commonly emerge and these are occasionally sufficiently severe that the FDA must change the labeling, append warnings to the package insert, or rarely withdraw the compound from the market. Phase IV trials or post-marketing studies provide an important opportunity to identify additional indications for use of the drug. These may be based on "off label" observations of the successful use of a compound in disorders related to the population testing in pivotal Phase III trials. For example, atypical antipsychotics were first developed for treatment of schizophrenia and have been tested in Phase IV programs to extend their indication to include bipolar mania (both acute and chronic phases) and bipolar depression. These expanded indications form an important part of the life-cycle management of a compound.

At the end of Phases III and IV, advances have been made in meeting the unmet need of the inadequately treated human disorder that stimulated the search for improved therapy (Figure 1). *Progress in Neurotherapeutics and Neuropsychopharmacology* will emphasize Phase II, III, and IV clinical trials and advances in clinical trial methodology. These are key translational research endeavors that link basic science observations of disease pathophysiology and mechanism of drug action to testing and establishment of efficacy in human clinical populations.

Neurologic and Psychiatric Therapeutics

Progress in Neurotherapeutics and Neuropsychopharmacology will include clinical trials and advances in clinical methodology involving compounds for the treatment of both primarily neurologic illnesses and psychotropic agents used for the treatment of idiopathic psychiatric disorders. Both neurologic and psychiatric conditions are included since it is obvious that successful intervention in a psychiatric disorder depends on modifying brain activity to minimize psychiatric symptoms. There is a spectrum of neuropsychopharmacologic intervention from purely symptomatic management of idiopathic psychiatric syndromes, to treatment of psychiatric disorders in patients who have neurologic disorders, to investigation and intervention in the emerging neurobiology of psychiatric conditions to treatment of identified pathophysiologic pathways in patients with neurologic disease (Figure 2).

There is increasing intellectual commerce between concepts of treatment of neurologic and psychiatric illnesses. For example, antidementia agents exhibit psychotropic properties and have beneficial effects on psychiatric aspects of Alzheimer's disease and other disorders (Emre *et al.*, 2004; Cummings, 2000). Similarly psychiatric compounds are increasingly recognized to exert neurologic effects. For example, the antidepressant properties of selective serotonin reuptake inhibitors correlate with their ability to produce neurogenesis in the hippocampus (Jacobs *et al.*, 2000). *Progress in Neurotherapeutics and Neuropsychopharmacology* will promote understanding of neurobiologic mechanisms and neuropsychotropic interventions by including clinical trials devoted to both neurologic and psychiatric syndromes.

Emerging Themes in Clinical Trials

Several major themes are emerging across clinical trials in neurologic and psychiatric disorders.

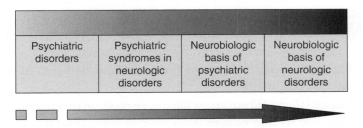

Fig. 2.
Relationship of neurotherapeutics and neuropsychopharmacology.

Informed Consent

Appropriate *informed consent* is difficult to achieve particularly in patients with neuropsychiatric illnesses that often alter judgment. Patients are desperate to have new treatments and clinicians are eager to advance therapeutic trials. Financial incentives involved in drug development further complicate the informed consent process. Means of insuring fully informed patient participants is an objective across clinical trials in all diseases.

Recruitment

Recruitment of appropriate patients in a timely manner falls short in many trials involving neurologic diseases. Despite a high prevalence of neurologic illnesses in the population, efficient screening, identification of patients that have all inclusion criteria and no exclusion criteria, and obtaining informed consent increasingly narrows the recruited population, delays trial completion, and impedes the emergence of new therapeutics. Establishment of community-based networks and community-based trial sites, reducing exclusionary criteria to allow the clinical trial population to more clearly mirror "real world" populations, and media campaigns to increase public awareness of neuropsychiatric illness and the need for clinical trials are methodologies that may improve recruitment. Increasing use of trial sites in Asia and India are anticipated.

Generalizability of Clinical Trial Results

Patients participating in clinical trials tend to be largely of Caucasian ethnicity and to be more highly educated, have better general physical health, have lower levels of psychopathology and are generally younger than unselected patient populations. These selection biases may influence the results of clinical trials and limit their generalizability. There are ethnic differences in drug metabolism which may go undetected using current clinical trial approaches.

There is an increased interest in conducting effectiveness trials in which the results of the current efficacy trials are extended into more typical patient populations using common clinical outcomes and trials conducted in community practices rather than specialized trial sites. Resource utilizations are an important outcome in effectiveness trials. These trials may provide new information on the performance of drugs when used in more "real world" settings.

Biomarkers

There is an increasing need for biomarkers that can be used as surrogate outcomes in clinical trials of disease-modifying agents. Clinical trial outcomes by themselves are unlikely to produce sufficient evidence of disease-modifying activity since it is difficult to distinguish symptomatic from disease-modifying effects on the basis

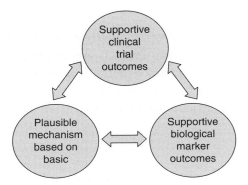

Fig. 3.
Relationship of clinical science, basic science and biomarkers in drug development and disease diagnosis.

of trial outcomes alone. Establishment of a drug as disease-modifying will require demonstration of a plausible mechanism of action in a basic science model, results from a clinical trial that are consistent with disease-modification, and effects on a surrogate biologic marker related to disease activity (Figure 3).

Progress is being made in the use of biologic markers in neurologic disorders. Positron emission tomography scans with amyloid ligands have evolved and promise to identify patients with Alzheimer's disease who have elevated levels of brain amyloid. These scans may function to monitor reduction of amyloid burden with effective therapeutic compounds (Klunk *et al.*, 2004).

Similarly measures of temporal lobe structures on magnetic resonance imaging (MRI) reflect progressive cerebral atrophy in neurodegenerative disorders such as Alzheimer's disease and slowing this rate of atrophy may function as a surrogate marker for the activity of a disease-modifying compound. Biologic markers relevant to other neurologic and psychiatric diseases are needed.

Treatment of Prodromal States

Identification and treatment of the earliest manifestations of neurologic and psychiatric illness is increasingly valued. Disease course is more difficult to modify and QOL more resistant to rescue when treatment is initiated after the brain disease is well established. For example, treatment of mild cognitive impairment with the aim of slowing the progression from this prodromal state to Alzheimer's disease is an increasingly important clinical trial strategy. Similarly, identification and treatment of the earliest phases of Parkinson's disease is a valuable clinical trial approach. The trial is terminated for the individual patient when treatment with initiation of levaodopa has become necessary and time to levaodopa therapy is the critical clinical trial measure. Treatment of prodromal phases of psychiatric illnesses, such as schizophrenia, are also of interest.

Disease Prevention

Primary prevention trials aimed at asymptomatic populations also deserve consideration. Prevention of stroke through control of stroke risk factors and amelioration of the progression from normal aging to mild cognitive impairment and Alzheimer's disease are important clinical trial paradigms. Identification of risk factors, some of which are modifiable, for neurologic and psychiatric illnesses will facilitate primary prevention trials.

Cross-Disease Treatment Approaches

Many neurologic disorders share common pathophysiologic mechanisms. Thus, inflammation is present in multiple sclerosis, stroke, and in neurodegenerative disorders, including Alzheimer's disease. Anti-inflammatory agents can possibly play a role in each of these conditions. Oxidative damage also is a common final pathway for cellular injury in many neurologic diseases. Excitotoxicity appears to play a role in both neurodegenerative and cerebrovascular diseases.

Neurodegenerative disorders are increasingly linked to protein misfolding and protein metabolism abnormalities (Cummings, 2003). Overproduction or accumulation of amyloid beta protein is regarded as the central even in Alzheimer's disease. Alpha synuclein is misfolded in idiopathic Parkinson's disease, tau and ubiquitin abnormalities are present in the frontotemporal lobar degeneration syndromes, huntingtin is abnormal in Huntington's disease, prion protein is accumulated abnormally in Creutzfeldt–Jakob disease, and other rare neurodegenerative disorders have their corresponding misfolded proteins. Information about how best to intervene in protein-misfolding disorders may result in principles applicable across many neurodegenerative disorders.

Pharmacogenomics

Both pharmacokinetic and pharmacodynamic responses have important genetic determinants. Increasing precision in pharmacogenomic studies may allow improved prediction of both efficacy and adverse responses to pharmacologic interventions. Pharmacogenomics may eventually provide a platform for developing highly individualized therapies that are best suited for the person's specific genetic constitution.

Pharmacoeconomics

Drug development occurs in a complex economic setting. Shareholders expect returns on investments in pharmaceutical and biotechnologic companies. New drugs must recoup the research costs of both successful and unsuccessful agents. Patients and drug purchasing organizations wish to minimize costs. Resource utilization is affected by effective drug treatment and these savings must be considered when calculating costs. Pharmacoeconomic outcomes are now more regularly included in clinical trials.

Quality of Life

There is greater interest in patient-centered outcomes that bear directly on the life of the patient and caregiver. The QOL measures of patient and caregiver are evolving and are included in some clinical trials as outcome assessments. QOL, health-related QOL, cost/benefit analyses, and quality-adjusted life years represent alternative current approaches to collecting patient-centered data. Those in a dearth of QOL instruments specifically useful in clinical trials that may be sensitive to drug–placebo differences.

Summary

Progress in Neurotherapeutics and Neuropsychopharmacology will bring together contributions from leading academic and industry investigators to provide a continuous update on pharmaceutic advances based on controlled clinical trials as well as advances in clinical trial methodology, including design, analysis, and use of biomarkers.

Disclosures

Dr. Cummings has served as a Consultant or performed research for AstraZeneca, Avanir, Eisai, Janssen, Lilly, Lundbeck, Memory, Merz, Neurochem, Novartis, Ono, Pfizer, *Takeda, Sanofi-Aventis, and Sepracor.

Acknowledgments

Dr. Cummings is supported by the National Institute on Aging (P50 AG 16570), the Alzheimer's Disease Research Centers of California and the Sidell-Kagan Foundation.

References

Cummings, J.L. (2000). Cholinesterase inhibitors: a new class of psychotropic compounds. *American Journal of Psychiatry*, 157, 4–15.

Cummings, J.L. (2003). Toward a molecular neuropsychiatry of neurodegenerative disease. *Annals of Neurology*, 54, 147–154.

Cummings, J.L. (2004). Alzheimer's disease. *New England Journal of Medicine*, 351, 56–67.

Emre, M., Aarsland, D., Albanese, A., *et al.* (2004). Rivastigmine for dementia associated with Parkinson's disease. *New England Journal of Medicine*, 351, 2509–2518.

Jacobs, B.L., Praag, H.V., Gage, F.H., *et al.* (2000). Adult brian neurogenesis and psychiatry: a novel theory of depression. *Molecular Psychiatry*, 5, 262–269.

Klunk, W.E., Engler, H., Nordberg, A., *et al.* (2004). Imaging brain amyloid in Alzheimer's disease with Pittsburgh compound-B. *Annals of Neurology*, 55, 306–319.

Lee, C.J., Lee, L.H., Lu, C., *et al.* (2003). *Development and Evaluation of Drugs* (2nd edn.). CRC Press, Boca Raton, Florida.

Ng, R. (2004). *Drugs from Discovery to Approval*. Wiley-Liss, Hoboken, New Jersey.

Progress in Neurotherapeutics and Neuropsychopharmacology, 1:1, 13–25 © 2006 Cambridge University Press
DOI: 10.1017/S1748232105000030   Printed in the United Kingdom

Rivastigmine in the Treatment of Dementia Associated with Parkinson's Disease: A Randomized, Double-blind, Placebo-controlled Study

---

Sibel Tekin and Roger Lane

Novartis Pharmaceuticals Corporation, East Hanover, NJ, USA; Email: sibel.tekin@novartis.com; roger.lane@novartis.com

Key words: Parkinson's disease; clinical trial; rivastigmine; executive function; cholinesterase inhibitor; dementia.

Introduction and Overview

Dementia is common in Parkinson's disease (PD), with an average prevalence of 40% (Cummings, 1988). The clinical phenotype of dementia associated with PD (PDD) is characterized by cognitive slowing, attentional, executive, and visuo-spatial dysfunction and memory impairment (Emre, 2003). PDD, also shares many clinical and pathological similarities with dementia with Lewy bodies (DLB) (McKeith *et al.*, 2004b).

Extensive Lewy body pathology is seen in the brainstem and neocortex in both DLB and PDD, in some cases with mild degrees of Alzheimer's disease (AD)-type pathology, and there is a pronounced loss of dopaminergic neurons in the substantia nigra (Esri & McShane, 1997). Recent studies using immunohisto-chemical staining techniques for identification of Lewy bodies show that in patients with PD, dementia correlates mostly with the presence of cortical and subcortical Lewy bodies – more so than with AD-like pathological changes (Braak *et al.*, 2005; Apaydin *et al.*, 2002). Lewy bodies are now known to be concomitant in a substantial proportion of AD patients and their presence is associated with faster cognitive and functional decline (Kraybill *et al.*, 2005; Jellinger, 2004). PDD and DLB are associated with marked cholinergic as well as dopaminergic deficits. Cholinergic deficits, which are generally more severe and more widespread than those seen in AD, are the most consistent neurochemical finding associated with cognitive and

Correspondence should be addressed to: Sibel Tekin, MD, Novartis Pharmaceuticals Corporation, One Health Plaza 59 Route 10, East Hanover NJ 07936, USA; Ph: +862 778 4242; Fax: +973 781 6550; Email: sibel.tekin@novartis.com.

neuropsychiatric symptoms of both PDD and DLB (Bohen *et al.*, 2003; Tiraboschi *et al.*, 2000; Perry *et al.*, 1985).

Patients with PDD have been excluded from previous clinical studies conducted with cholinesterase inhibitors (ChE-Is) in AD due to the presence of underlying PD. Therefore, a large randomized, double-blind, placebo-controlled study was performed to evaluate the efficacy and safety of rivastigmine versus placebo for 24 weeks in patients with PDD.

Rivastigmine: Pharmacology and Relevant Past Experience

Rivastigmine is a slowly reversible, brain-selective inhibitor of acetylcholinesterase (AChE) and butyrylcholinesterase (BuChE) that shows selectivity for forms of these enzymes found in areas of the brain affected by neurodegeneration (Geula *et al.*, 2004; Enz *et al.*, 1993; Enz & Bodekke, 1991). Rivastigmine has demonstrated favorable efficacy and safety in patients with dementia of the Alzheimer-type (Anand *et al.*, 2000; Rösler *et al.*, 1999; Corey-Bloom *et al.*, 1998), and is widely approved for the treatment of mild to moderate AD.

Rivastigmine also demonstrated benefits in a multi-center, placebo-controlled, double-blind, 20-week study in 120 patients with DLB (McKeith *et al.*, 2000). Rivastigmine 6–12 mg/day provided significant beneficial effects on cognitive change, behavioral symptoms and attention deficits compared with placebo (Wesnes *et al.*, 2002; McKeith *et al.*, 2000). Behavioral benefits included those that were particularly relevant to DLB: apathy, indifference, anxiety, delusions, hallucinations, and aberrant motor behavior, including nocturnal wandering (McKeith *et al.*, 2000). In a *post hoc* analysis, the presence of hallucinations at baseline, in 74% of patients, was associated with markedly greater responses on attention than in patients without this symptom at baseline (McKeith *et al.*, 2004a). An open-label extension of this 20-week study ($n = 29$) suggested that cognitive and behavioral benefits were sustained for at least 96 weeks (Grace *et al.*, 2001).

Preliminary studies of rivastigmine in PDD also suggested significant cognitive and behavioral benefits (Fogelson *et al.*, 2003; Bullock & Cameron, 2002; Loos *et al.*, 2002; Reading, *et al.*, 2001; Van Laar *et al.*, 2001). Rivastigmine did not seem to be associated with persistent worsening extra-pyramidal parkinsonian symptoms, although tremor was infrequently reported.

Clinical Trial

Subjects

The multi-center, double-blind, placebo-controlled EXPRESS (Exelon in Patients with PDD) study was conducted between 2002 and 2004. Patients were recruited from clinical and research centers in Austria, Belgium, Canada, France, Germany,

Italy, The Netherlands, Norway, Portugal, Spain, Turkey, and the UK. They were males or females of at least 50-years old with a diagnosis of PD according to the UK PD Society Brain Bank clinical diagnostic criteria (Gibb & Lees, 1988), and PDD according to the 4th edition of the *Diagnostic and Statistical Manual of Mental Disorders* (DSM-IV) (American Psychiatric Association, 1994). Patients had mild to moderately severe dementia as defined by a Mini-Mental State Examination (MMSE) score of 10–24, with the onset of dementia symptoms occurring at least 2 years after the first diagnosis of idiopathic PD.

Trial Methods

Patients were randomly assigned to double-blind treatment for 24 weeks with rivastigmine (3–12 mg/day) or placebo in an assignment ratio of 2 : 1. Treatment was started with 3 mg/day of rivastigmine or placebo. Doses were escalated at a minimum of 4-week intervals (3 mg/day steps at each interval) during a 16-week dose-escalation phase. The highest well-tolerated dose (maximum 12 mg/day) for each individual patient was maintained for the rest of the study, although dose adjustments were permitted in case of adverse events (AEs) or any other problems. Efficacy assessments were completed at baseline and weeks 16 (completion of titration phase) and 24.

Following the double-blind trial, all patients (irrespective of their double-blind treatment) were permitted to enter an open-label extension study, during which they received rivastigmine 3–12 mg/day for a further 24 weeks.

Outcome Measures

Primary efficacy measures were the Alzheimer's Disease Assessment Scale-cognitive subscale (ADAS-cog) (Rosen *et al.*, 1984) and the Alzheimer's Disease Cooperative Study–Clinician's Global Impression of Change (ADCS-CGIC) (Schneider *et al.*, 1997). Secondary efficacy measures were the Alzheimer's Disease Cooperative Study–Activities of Daily Living (ADCS-ADL) scale (Galasko *et al.*, 1997), Ten-item NeuroPsychiatric Inventory (NPI-10) (Cummings *et al.*, 1994), Mini-Mental State Examination (MMSE) (Folstein *et al.*, 1975), Cognitive Drug Research (CDR) Computerized Assessment System Power of Attention test (Simpson *et al.*, 1991), and the Delis–Kaplan Executive Function System (D-KEFS) verbal fluency test (Delis *et al.*, 2001) and Ten-Point Clock–Drawing test (Manos & Wu, 1994) for the assessment of executive functions.

Safety evaluations included recording all AEs, laboratory tests, electrocardiogram results, and vital signs and body weight. Changes in motor function and symptoms of parkinsonism were assessed with the motor examination section of the Unified Parkinson's Disease Rating Scale (UPDRS part III) (Fahn *et al.*, 1987) at baseline and weeks 16 and 24.

Analysis

Patients who had at least one dose of study medication, and at least one safety evaluation post-baseline, were considered for safety analysis. The primary population for efficacy analyses was defined as the intent-to-treat with retrieved dropout (ITT–RDO) population, comprising all randomized patients who received at least one dose of study medication and had at least a baseline and post-baseline assessment for one of the primary efficacy variables. RDO patients discontinued treatment early but continued to attend scheduled visits for efficacy evaluations.

The main ITT–RDO data from the double-blind study have been published previously (Emre *et al.*, 2004). Here, we also show data for the additional analyses specified in the protocol that were considered supportive to the main analysis: ITT-last observation carried forward (LOCF; randomized patients with at least one primary efficacy assessment while being treated), and observed cases (OC; randomized patients who had evaluations on treatment at designated assessment times, with no imputation of missing values).

For the double-blind study, changes from baseline on the ADAS-cog were assessed by analysis of covariance (ANCOVA), with baseline values as covariates, and treatment and countries as factors. The main ADCS–CGIC analysis was the treatment comparison based on a Cochran–Mantel–Haenszel (CMH) test. Secondary efficacy variables were analyzed using either an ANCOVA model with treatment, country, and the corresponding baseline measurement as covariates (for continuous variables), or a CMH test (for categorical variables).

For the additional 24-week open-label treatment extension, the OC population was used (to minimize bias from early discontinuations over the long-term treatment period). Only summary statistics were performed on efficacy variables due to the uncontrolled, open-label nature of this phase of the study.

Results

In total, 541 patients were randomized to rivastigmine or placebo. Baseline demographic and background characteristics have been published previously (Emre *et al.*, 2004). The mean age of the study population was 72.7 years, and 35.1% of patients were females. The mean baseline MMSE score was 19.3. No significant differences between the two groups were observed with regard to baseline characteristics; 501 patients were available for the ITT–RDO efficacy analysis, and 449 were available for the LOCF and OC efficacy analyses. The mean dose of rivastigmine was 8.6 mg/day at the end of the dose escalation phase, and this dose remained stable throughout the maintenance phase (Emre *et al.*, 2004).

Patients receiving rivastigmine showed consistent, statistically significant improvements compared with patients receiving placebo at week 24 with respect to ADAS-cog and ADCS-CGIC scores in all efficacy populations (Table 1). Rivastigmine provided consistent, statistically significant benefits over placebo

Table 1. **Results of the Primary Efficacy Variables**

	BASELINE SCORE		CHANGE AT WEEK 16		CHANGE AT WEEK 24		24 WEEK BETWEEN GROUP DIFFERENCE
	n	MEAN (SD)	*n*	MEAN (SD)	*n*	MEAN (SD)	
ADAS-cog							
ITT–RDO							
Rivastigmine	329	23.8 (10.2)	329	2.3 (7.3)	329	2.1 (8.2)	2.9[a]
Placebo	161	24.3 (10.5)	161	0.3 (6.5)	161	−0.7 (7.5)	$p < 0.001$
LOCF							
Rivastigmine	287	24.0 (10.3)	287	2.8 (7.4)	287	2.5 (8.4)	3.5[a]
Placebo	154	24.5 (10.6)	154	0.3 (6.7)	154	−0.8 (7.5)	$p < 0.001$
OC							
Rivastigmine	284	23.9 (10.3)	284	2.8 (7.4)	256	2.9 (8.3)	3.8[a]
Placebo	150	24.5 (10.6)	150	0.3 (6.8)	139	−1.0 (7.6)	$p < 0.001$
ADCS-CGIC							
ITT–RDO							
Rivastigmine	–	–	318	3.8 (1.4)	329	3.8 (1.4)	0.5
Placeebo	–	–	159	4.1 (1.4)	165	4.3 (1.5)	$p = 0.007$
LOCF							
Rivastigmine	–	–	282	3.6 (1.3)	289	3.7 (1.4)	0.6
Placebo	–	–	153	4.1 (1.4)	158	4.3 (1.5)	$p < 0.001$
OC							
Rivastigmine	–	–	282	3.6 (1.3)	252	3.7 (1.4)	0.5
Placebo	–	–	153	4.1 (1.4)	145	4.2 (1.5)	$p < 0.001$

ADAS-cog: Alzheimer's Disease Assessment Scale-cognitive subscale; ADCS-CGIC: Alzheimer's Disease Cooperative Study–Clinician's Global Impression of Change (there are no baseline scores for the ADCS-CGIC because there was no comparator at baseline on which to base an impression of change).
[a] Difference between changes from baseline calculated based on Least Squares Means from the ANCOVA model.

($p < 0.05$) at 24 weeks on the ADCS–ADL, NPI-10, MMSE, and CDR in all populations, except for the OC result on the NPI-10, which did not reach statistical significance (Figures 1–4). Executive function tests were performed only at selected sites so OC analyses only were provided for these parameters; statistically significant benefits over placebo were seen (Emre *et al.*, 2004).

Three hundred and thirty-four patients were elected to enter the 24-week open-label extension (Poewe *et al.* (in press)). Upon switching to rivastigmine, patients in the original placebo group experienced a 2.8-point improvement in their ADAS-cog scores between weeks 24 and 48. This improvement was of a similar magnitude to that seen in the original rivastigmine double-blind group during weeks 0–24. Second, patients who received double-blind rivastigmine followed by open-label rivastigmine (giving a total treatment duration of 48 weeks), on average, were still improved by 2 points above week 0 baseline levels at week 48. Treatment benefits were sustained on the ADCS-ADL, NPI-10, D-KEFS verbal fluency test, and MMSE, for up to 48 weeks.

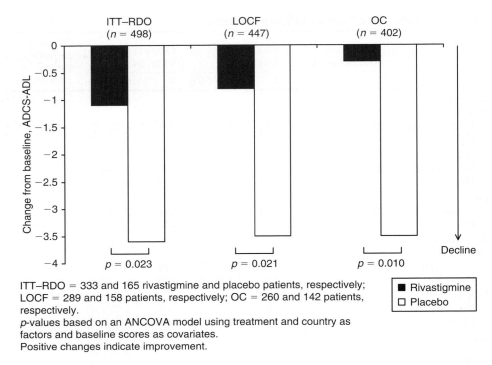

ITT–RDO = 333 and 165 rivastigmine and placebo patients, respectively;
LOCF = 289 and 158 patients, respectively; OC = 260 and 142 patients,
respectively.
p-values based on an ANCOVA model using treatment and country as
factors and baseline scores as covariates.
Positive changes indicate improvement.

Fig. 1.
Changes from baseline after 24 weeks on the ADCS-ADL (ITT–RDO, LOCF, OC).

Tolerability and Safety

The most common AEs during the double-blind study (weeks 1–24) were nausea
and vomiting (29.0% versus 11.2% nausea, and 16.6% versus 1.7% vomiting, in
the rivastigmine versus placebo groups, respectively) (Emre *et al.*, 2004). Most
AEs were mild or moderate. The occurrence of serious AEs was similar in both the
treatment groups (rivastigmine 13.0% and placebo 14.5%). A total of 131 patients
(27.3% rivastigmine and 17.9% placebo) discontinued the double-blind study
prematurely. AEs contributing to the greater discontinuation rate in the rivastigmine
group included nausea (causing 3.6% and 0.6% of patients to withdraw from the
rivastigmine and placebo groups, respectively), vomiting (1.9% and 0.6%), and
tremor (1.7% and 0.0%). When all AEs that may potentially have been associated
with worsening PD were combined, the incidence rate was higher in patients on
rivastigmine (27.3%) than on placebo (15.6%). Tremor was the most commonly
reported AE potentially associated with PD. In a *post hoc* analysis, maximal incidence of these events was seen during the dose-escalation phase, and they decreased
to levels comparable with the placebo group during the maintenance phase (data
on file, Novartis Pharma, AG). Furthermore, these events were not associated with

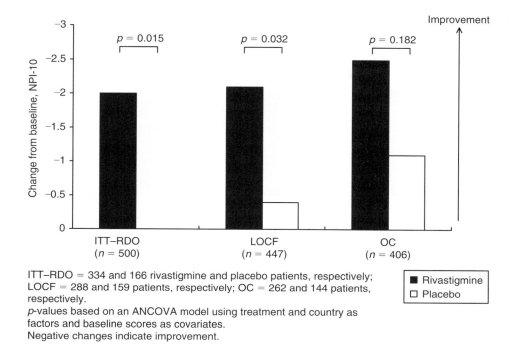

ITT–RDO = 334 and 166 rivastigmine and placebo patients, respectively;
LOCF = 288 and 159 patients, respectively; OC = 262 and 144 patients,
respectively.
p-values based on an ANCOVA model using treatment and country as
factors and baseline scores as covariates.
Negative changes indicate improvement.

Fig. 2.
Changes from baseline after 24 weeks on the NPI-10 (ITT–RDO, LOCF, OC).

episodes of nausea or vomiting that could have interrupted compliance with dopaminergic medications that the patients were receiving. During the double-blind core study, the mean doses of L-DOPA and dopamine agonists remained stable in both the rivastigmine and placebo groups. Increases in doses, or new introduction of anti-psychotics were more frequent in the placebo group (increased in 2.5% of rivastigmine and 3.9% of placebo groups; newly introduced in 7.7% and 11.2%, respectively). The UPDRS motor ratings, which were evaluated at the end of the titration phase (week 16) and at study endpoint, did not reveal significantly different effects of rivastigmine versus placebo ($p = 0.83$), including changes in tremor sub-items ($p = 0.84$) (Emre *et al.*, 2004).

Similarly, after the start of open-label rivastigmine treatment (weeks 25–48), predominant AEs were nausea (18.6%) and vomiting (11.1%) (Poewe *et al.* (in press)). Most AEs were mild or moderate; 17.1% of patients reported serious AEs. Overall, 11.4% of patients withdrew from the open-label extension due to AEs (including deaths), most frequently due to nausea and vomiting. Any worsening or occurrence of parkinsonian symptoms as AEs was not reflected by UPDRS motor scores, which remained relatively constant over the course of the 48-week study.

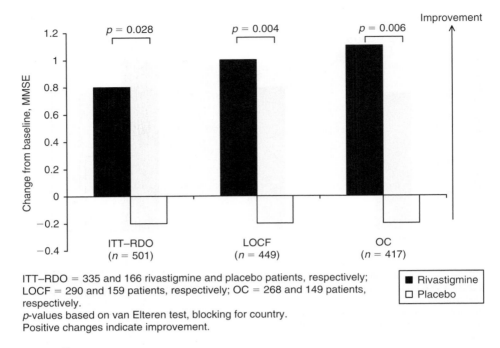

ITT–RDO = 335 and 166 rivastigmine and placebo patients, respectively;
LOCF = 290 and 159 patients, respectively; OC = 268 and 149 patients,
respectively.
p-values based on van Elteren test, blocking for country.
Positive changes indicate improvement.

Fig. 3.
Changes from baseline after 24 weeks on the MMSE (ITT–RDO, LOCF, OC).

No clinically significant changes in vital signs were reported. ECG analysis did not reveal clinically significant abnormalities with rivastigmine treatment, except for rare incidences of bradycardia. No new safety or tolerability problems emerged with long-term rivastigmine treatment. There were 11 deaths during the double-blind phase (4 of 362 patients [1.1%] in the rivastigmine group, 7 of 179 [3.9%] in the placebo group) (Emre *et al.*, 2004), and 7 [2.1%] during the open-label extension (Poewe *et al.* (in press)).

Unique Aspects of Trial

This is the first large-scale, randomized, double-blind, placebo-controlled, multi-center study demonstrating significant benefits of a ChE-I in PDD to be completed and published.

Seventy-six percent of the total study population completed the double-blind study. Failure to obtain information at the final visit for some of the patients who discontinued the study prematurely may limit the interpretation of these results. Nevertheless, results from the three populations used for the statistical analyses (ITT–RDO, LOCF, OC), two of which used imputations for early withdrawals,

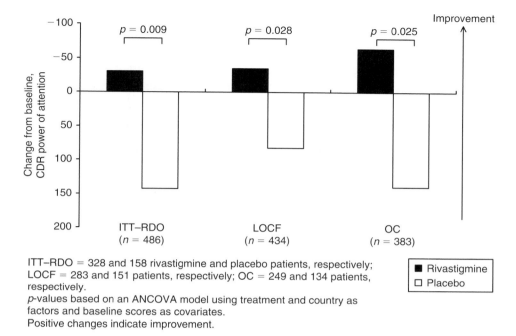

ITT–RDO = 328 and 158 rivastigmine and placebo patients, respectively; LOCF = 283 and 151 patients, respectively; OC = 249 and 134 patients, respectively.

p-values based on an ANCOVA model using treatment and country as factors and baseline scores as covariates.

Positive changes indicate improvement.

Fig. 4.
Changes from Baseline after 24 Weeks on the CDR Power of Attention Measure (ITT–RDO, LOCF, OC).

provided consistent findings, implying that attrition rate did not confound the interpretation of the study outcome.

To differentiate them from DLB patients, the patients taking part in this study were carefully selected with at least a 2-year delay (mean 6.8 years) between the diagnosis of PD and the onset of symptoms of dementia, and their dementia profile was predetermined to meet the DSM-IV criteria for a diagnosis of PDD. A range of concomitant illnesses and medications were permitted. The baseline characteristics of patients showed that patients had prominent deficits in attention and executive functioning in addition to memory problems (Emre *et al.*, 2004), differing from the typical clinical characteristics of mild to moderate AD (Rosenstein, 1998). *Post hoc* analyses of the double-blind trial showed that significant benefits of rivastigmine over placebo were seen on all aspects of attention assessed: sustained attention, focused attention, consistence of responding, and central-processing speed (Wesnes *et al.*, 2005).

Conclusions

Rivastigmine in daily doses of 3–12 mg (mean dose 8.6 mg) produced statistically significant and clinically relevant improvements in patients with mild to moderate

PDD. Compared with placebo, patients given rivastigmine experienced better global ratings, improvements in cognition, including executive functioning and attention, and in behavioral symptoms, indicating significant benefits in all key symptom domains. The clinical relevance was reflected in the improvement of activities of daily living. The observed effect sizes on the ADAS-cog were similar to those observed in AD patients treated with ChE-Is (Bryant *et al.*, 2001; Doody *et al.*, 2001).

Rivastigmine was well tolerated in this patient population. Serious AEs did not differ between the groups. Rivastigmine was not associated with any clinically relevant change in laboratory tests, vital signs, or electrocardiogram results. Adverse events and discontinuations for centrally mediated gastrointestinal cholinergic effects of nausea and vomiting were lower than those seen in previous studies of rivastigmine in AD (Anand *et al.*, 2000; Rösler *et al.*, 1999; Corey-Bloom *et al.*, 1998), possibly reflecting the slower dose escalation in this study or a reduced likelihood of these events in PDD patients. Worsening of parkinsonian symptoms, mainly of tremor, was more frequently reported in rivastigmine-treated patients; but these were dose-titration related, usually transient, rarely severe, and infrequently resulted in withdrawal from the study. Moreover, these reports were not supported by changes in overall or individual item of UPDRS motor scale assessments at week 16 and at study termination, compared with baseline or placebo.

In conclusion, this is the first large placebo-controlled study to demonstrate the efficacy of an intervention targeting PDD (Emre *et al.*, 2004; Poewe *et al.* (in press)). These findings support those of a previous multi-center, placebo-controlled study of rivastigmine in DLB (McKeith *et al.*, 2000), a condition that shares many clinical and pathological features with PDD. Rivastigmine has been shown to provide significant improvements in key symptom domains of these two Lewy body dementias, and was generally well tolerated. Dementia is a major prognostic factor for progressive disability and nursing home placement in patients with PDD or DLB, and the current findings may have important implications for clinical practice.

Influence on the Field

No other agents have proven efficacy in PDD or DLB in large, randomized, double-blind studies, and there are currently no approved treatments for these dementia types. The findings of the study indicate that the use of rivastigmine in patients with dementia associated with PD has a similar safety profile as in patients with AD, and provided significant improvements in cognition, executive functioning, activities of daily living, behavior, attention, and global functioning.

References

American Psychiatric Association. (1994). *Diagnostic and Statistical Manual of Mental Disorders*, 4th edn. Washington DC: American Psychiatric Association.

Anand, R., Messina, J., & Hartman, R. (2000). Dose-response effect of rivastigmine in the treatment of Alzheimer's disease. *International Journal of Geriatrics Psychopharmacology*, 2, 68–72.

Apaydin, H., Ahlskog, J.E., Parisi, J.E., Boeve, B.F., & Dickson, D.W. (2002). Parkinson disease neuropathology: later-developing dementia and loss of the levodopa response. *Archives of Neurology*, 59, 102–112.

Bohnen, N.I., Kaufer, D.I., Ivanco, L.S., et al. (2003). Cortical cholinergic function is more severely affected in parkinsonian dementia than in Alzheimer disease: an in vivo positron emission tomographic study. *Archives of Neurology*, 60, 1745–1748.

Braak, H., Rub, U., Jansen Steur, E.N., Del Tredici, K., & de Vos, R.A. (2005). Cognitive status correlates with neuropathologic stage in Parkinson disease. *Neurology*, 64, 1404–1410.

Bryant, J., Clegg, A., Nicholson, T., et al. (2001). Clinical and cost-effectiveness of donepezil, rivastigmine and galantamine for Alzheimer's disease: a rapid and systematic review. *Health Technology Assessments*, 5, 1–137.

Bullock, R., & Cameron, A. (2002). Rivastigmine for the treatment of dementia and visual hallucinations associated with Parkinson's disease. *Current Medical Research and Opinion*, 18, 258–264.

Corey-Bloom, J., Anand, R., & Veach, J. (1998). A randomized trial evaluating the efficacy and safety of ENA 713 (rivastigmine tartrate), a new acetylcholinesterase inhibitor, in patients with mild to moderately severe Alzheimer's disease. *International Journal of Geriatrics Psychopharmacology*, 1, 55–65.

Cummings, J.L. (1988). Intellectual impairment in Parkinson's disease: clinical, pathologic, and biochemical correlates. *Journal of Geriatric Psychiatry Neurology*, 1, 24–36.

Cummings, J.L., Mega, M., Gray, K., et al. (1994). The neuropsychiatric inventory: comprehensive assessment of psychopathology in dementia. *Neurology*, 44, 2308–2314.

Delis, D.C., Kaplan, E., & Kramer, J.H. (2001). Delis–Kaplan Executive Function System. Texas: Psychological Corporation.

Doody, R.S., Stevens, J.C., Beck, C., et al. (2001). Practice parameter: management of dementia (an evidence-based review). Report of the Quality Standards Subcommittee of the American Academy of Neurology. *Neurology*, 56, 1154–1166.

Emre, M. (2003). Dementia associated with Parkinson's disease. *Lancet Neurology*, 3, 229–237.

Emre, M., Aarsland, D., Albanese, A., et al. (2004). Rivastigmine for the dementia associated with Parkinson's disease. *New England Journal of Medicine*, 351, 29–38.

Enz, A., & Bodekke, H. (1991). Pharmacologic and clinicopharmacologic properties of SDZ ENA 713, a centrally selective acetylcholinesterase inhibitor. *Annals of the New York Academy of Sciences*, 640, 272–275.

Enz, A., Amstutz, R., Boddeke, H., Gmelin, G., & Malanowski, J. (1993). Brain selective inhibition of acetylcholinesterase: a novel approach to therapy for Alzheimer's disease. *Progress in Brain Research*, 98, 431–438.

Esiri, M.M., & McShane, R.H. (1997). In: Esiri, M.M., Morris, J.H. (eds.), *The Neuropathology of Dementia*. Cambridge, UK: Cambridge University Press.

Fahn, S., Elton, R.L., & Members of the UPDRS development committee. (1987). Unified Parkinson's disease rating scale. In: Fahn, S., Marsden, C.D., Calne, D.B., Goldstein, M. (eds.), *Recent Developments in Parkinson's Disease*. Florham Park, NJ: MacMillan Healthcare Information, pp. 153–164.

Fogelson, N., Kogan, E., Korczyn, A.D., et al. (2003). Effects of rivastigmine on the quantitative EEG in demented Parkinsonian patients. *Acta Neurological Scandinavica*, 107, 252–255.

Folstein, M.F., Folstein, F.E., & McHugh, P.R. (1975). "Mini-mental" state. A practical method for grading the cognitive state of patients for the clinician. *Journal of Psychiatric Research*, 12, 189–198.

Galasko, D., Bennett, D., Sano, M., *et al.* (1997). An inventory to assess activities of daily living for clinical trials in Alzheimer's disease. The Alzheimer's Disease Cooperative Study. *Alzheimer Disease and Associated Disorders*, 11 (Suppl. 2), S33–S39.

Geula, C., Eskander, M., Atkinson, L., *et al.* (2004). Rivastigmine is a potent inhibitor of cholinesterases in plaques and tangles. Poster presented at the American Psychiatric Association Annual Meeting, New York, 1–6 May 2004.

Gibb, W.R., & Lees, A.J. (1988). The relevance of the Lewy body to the pathogenesis of idiopathic Parkinson's disease. *Journal of Neurology Neurosurgery and Psychiatry*, 51, 745–752.

Grace, J., Daniel, S., Stevens, T., *et al.* (2001). Long-term use of rivastigmine in patients with dementia with Lewy bodies: an open-label trial. *International Psychogeriatrics*, 13, 199–205.

Jellinger, K.A. (2004). Lewy body-related alpha-synucleinopathy in the aged human brain. *Journal of Neural Transmission*, 111, 1219–1235.

Kraybill, M.L., Larson, E.B., Tsuang, D.W., *et al.* (2005). Cognitive differences in dementia patients with autopsy-verified AD, Lewy body pathology, or both. *Neurology*, 64, 2069–2073.

Loos, C., Wenig, M., & Steinwachs, C. (2002). Rivastigmine is effective and well tolerated in the treatment of parkinsonian psychosis of geriatric patients. Poster presented at the 6th Congress of the European Federation of Neurological Sciences, Vienna, Austria, 26–29 October 2002.

Manos, P.J., & Wu, R. (1994). The ten point clock test: a quick screen and grading method for cognitive impairment in medical and surgical patients. *International Journal of Psychiatry in Medicine*, 24, 229–244.

McKeith, I., Del Ser, T., Spano, P.-F., *et al.* (2000). Efficacy of rivastigmine in dementia with Lewy bodies: a randomised, double blind, placebo-controlled international study. *Lancet*, 356, 2031–2036.

McKeith, I.G., Wesnes, K.A., Perry, E., & Ferrara, R. (2004a). Hallucinations predict attentional improvements with rivastigmine in dementia with Lewy bodies. *Dementia and Geriatric Cognitive Disorders*, 18, 94–100.

McKeith, I., Mintzer, J., Aarsland, D., *et al.* (2004b). Dementia with Lewy bodies. *Lancet Neurology*, 3, 19–28.

Perry, E.K., Curtis, M., Dick, D.J., *et al.* (1985). Cholinergic correlates of cognitive impairment in Parkinson's disease: comparison with Alzheimer's disease. *Journal of Neurology Neurosurgery and Psychiatry*, 48, 413–421.

Poewe, W., Wolters, E., Emre, M., *et al.* (2005). Long-term benefits of rivastigmine in dementia associated with Parkinson's disease: an active treatment extension study. *Movement disorders*, 14 October, published online (Google: Journal of movement disorders).

Reading, P.J., Luce, A.K., & McKeith, I.G. (2001). Rivastigmine in the treatment of parkinsonian psychosis and cognitive impairment: preliminary findings from an open trial. *Movement Disorders*, 16, 1171–1195.

Rosen, W.G., Mohs, R.C., & Davis, K.L. (1984). A new rating scale for Alzheimer's disease. *American Journal of Psychiatry*, 141, 1356–1364.

Rosenstein, L.D. (1998). Differential diagnosis of the major progressive dementias and depression in middle and late adulthood: a summary of the literature of the early 1990s. *Neuropsychology Review*, 8, 109–167.

Rösler, M., Anand, R., Cicin-Sain, A., *et al.* (1999). Efficacy and safety of rivastigmine in patients with Alzheimer's disease: international randomised controlled trial. *British Medical Journal*, 318, 633–640.

Schneider, L.S., Olin, J.T., Doody, R.S., *et al.* (1997). Validity and reliability of the Alzheimer's disease cooperative study – clinical global impression of Change. The Alzheimer's Disease Cooperative Study. *Alzheimer Disease and Associated Disorders*, 11 (Suppl. 2), S22–S32.

Simpson, P.M., Surmon, D.J., Wesnes, K.A., & Wilcock, G.K. (1991). The cognitive drug research computerized assessment system for demented patients: a validation study. *International Journal of Geriatric Psychiatry*, 6, 95–102.

Tiraboschi, P., Hansen, L.A., Alford, M., *et al.* (2000). Cholinergic dysfunction in diseases with Lewy bodies. *Neurology*, 54, 407–411.

Van Laar, T., de Vries, J.J., Nakhosteen, A., & Leenders, K.L. (2001). Rivastigmine is effective and safe as anti-psychotic treatment in patients with Parkinson's disease. Poster presented at the 13th International Congress on Parkinson's Disease, Helsinki, Finland, July 2001.

Wesnes, K., McKeith, I.G., Ferrara, R., *et al.* (2002). Effects of rivastigmine on cognitive function in dementia with Lewy bodies: a randomised placebo-controlled international study using the cognitive drug research computerised assessment system. *Dementia and Geriatric Cognitive Disorders*, 13, 183–192.

Wesnes, K.A., McKeith, I., Edgar, C., *et al.* (2005). Benefits of rivastigmine on attention in dementia associated with PD. *Neurology*, 65: 1654–1656.

Progress in Neurotherapeutics and Neuropsychopharmacology, 1:1, 27–36 © 2006 Cambridge University Press
DOI: 10.1017/S1748232105000042   Printed in the United Kingdom

Modafinil for the Treatment of Fatigue in Multiple Sclerosis

Bruno Stankoff

Centre d'Investigation Clinique, Hopital Pitié-Salpêtrière, Paris, France; Service de Pharmacologie, Hopital Pitié-Salpêtrière, Paris, France; Email:bruno.stankoff@psl.ap-hop-paris.fr

Catherine Lubetzki

Fédération de Neurologie, Hopital Pitié-Salpêtrière, Paris, France; Email:catherine.lubetzki@psl.ap-hop-paris.fr

Michel Clanet

Fédération de Neurologie, CHU de Toulouse, France; Email:clanet@cict.fr

Key words: Multiple sclerosis; modafinil; fatigue; neurotherapeutics; clinical trial.

Introduction and Overview

Fatigue is a disabling symptom in multiple sclerosis (MS), affecting more than 50% of patients with the diagnostic of clinically definite MS. Among patients with fatigue, a high proportion indicates that it represents the most troublesome symptom of the disease (Fisk *et al.*, 1994). As fatigue is a subjective feeling, it usually receives little attention from physicians, patients' family and employers, whereas it has a tremendous impact on the activities of daily life, interfering with work, family life and social activities.

The diagnosis and management of fatigue in MS are complicated by number of issues, including the many forms that the symptom can take. In some cases fatigue may be related to depression, cognitive dysfunction, poor sleeping or motor impairment, defining secondary fatigue. Nevertheless, for many patients, fatigue exists independently of both motor weakness, cognitive or mood disorders: this primary fatigue is felt as an overwhelming sense of tiredness, a lack of energy or a feeling of exhaustion; patients also have the feeling that the effort required to perform action is disproportionately high, and, as a consequence, tend to reduce their physical activity (Comi *et al.*, 2001). This fatigue affects mood and the ability to

Correspondence should be addressed to: Bruno Stankoff, Centre d'Investigation Clinique, Hopital Pitié-Salpêtrière, Paris, France; Email: bruno.stankoff@psl.ap-hop-paris.fr.

cope with the disease (Ritvo *et al.*, 1996), and decreases the quality of life (Schwartz *et al.*, 1996).

The pathophysiology of fatigue in MS remains poorly understood, despite the multiplicity of putative mechanisms that have been considered (Comi *et al.*, 2001): muscle and motor disorders; conduction block along demyelinated axons which could be facilitated by increased body temperature or by repetitive firing of neurons; cytokine dyregulation; neuro-endocrine disorders; reduction in brain metabolic activity in some areas (prefrontal cortex, premotor cortex, putamen, right supplementary area) (Roelcke *et al.*, 1997); impaired interaction between functionally-related cortical and subcortical areas (Filippi *et al.*, 2002).

The lack of knowledge about the pathophysiology of fatigue largely explains the poor efficacy of the drugs currently used. The most usual treatment options include amantadine, pemoline, 4-aminopyridine, 3,4-aminopyridine and serotonin reuptake inhibitors (SRIs): excepted for SRIs that have not been evaluated in well-designed trials for this indication, most molecules were able to provide only limited benefit among subgroups of patients. For instance, studies of amantadine have shown that only 20–40% of MS patients could experience mild short-term reduction in fatigue (Krupp *et al.*, 1995; Cohen *et al.*, 1989; the Canadian MS research group, 1987; Murray *et al.*, 1985). For pemoline, one clinical trial has shown a possible benefit with high dose (75 mg/day) (Weinshenker *et al.*, 1992), whereas another trial failed to show any efficacy at 56.25 mg/day (Krupp *et al.*, 1995). 4-aminopyridine has shown some benefit for neurological symptoms such as motor weakness, ambulation and fatigue (Rossini *et al.*, 2001; Bever *et al.*, 1994; Polman *et al.*, 1994a; Van Diemen *et al.*, 1992). The related molecule, 3,4-diaminopyridine is better tolerated, but its efficacy on fatigue still has to be demonstrated (Sheean *et al.*, 1998; Bever *et al.*, 1996; Polman *et al.*, 1994b).

Purpose of the Study

The purpose of this trial was to evaluate the efficacy of modafinil (200–400 mg/day), compared to placebo, for the short-term treatment of fatigue among MS patients in a double-blind parallel group study.

Agent

Modafinil is a wake-promoting agent aimed at alleviating excessive daytime sleepiness in patients with narcolepsy, obstructive sleep apnea syndrome, and shift work sleep disorder (Banerjee *et al.*, 2004).

The brain target of modafinil, as well as its precise mechanism of action, still remain uncertain, despite it has been reported to act mainly in the hypothalamic area by modulating noradrenergic, dopaminergic, and gabaergique neurotransmission (Wisor & Eriksson, 2005; Scammell *et al.*, 2000; Lin *et al.*, 1996). Compared to other psychostimulants such as amphetamines, or methylphenidate, modafinil has little abuse potential. However, euphoric and psychoactive effect have been described, especially at high dose and among subjects experienced with drugs of abuse.

Recently, modafinil has been evaluated in two pilot clinical trials for its ability to improve MS fatigue (Rammohan *et al.*, 2002; Zifko *et al.*, 2002). There were no major safety concern, and both studies suggested a clinical benefit with lower doses than those required in narcolepsy. Nevertheless, one study had an open-label design (Zifko *et al.*, 2002) the other was only single blind (Rammohan *et al.*, 2002), and there was a need for a larger double-blind placebo-controlled study.

Clinical Trial

Subjects

Men and women, 18–65 years of age (inclusive), suffering from MS according to Poser criteria, and complaining of chronic fatigue for at least 6 months with a global score on the Modified Fatigue Impact Scale (MFIS) ⩾45 were enrolled in the study between May, 2001 and December, 2001. The EDSS score had to be between 0 and 6.5 (inclusive). Exclusion criteria were as follows: relapse or steroid course within the 2 months before randomization; women that were pregnant, breast-feeding, or not using an adequate method of contraception; uncontrolled seizures; depressive disorder (attested by the Montgomery/Asberg Depression Rating Scale, MADRS score ⩾20); anxiety (attested by the Covi Anxiety Scale, CAS score ⩾3); dementia.

Disease modifying therapy with beta interferon, gatiramer acetate, azathioprin or methotrexate were admitted but had to be stabilized at a fixed dose for at least 6 months. Every symptomatic treatment for fatigue had to be withdrawn at least 14 days before randomization.

Sample Size

We have fixed the minimal pertinent difference between the two groups on the MFIS at 15, which was consistent with the preliminary results obtained in a group of eight patients who had undergone compassionate treatment with modafinil for 1 month. For this group of patients the standard deviation was 22 for the MFIS score. Assuming a type-1 error rate of 5%, and a study power of 90%, the number of patients required per group was 45. Considering that 20% of patients could be lost of follow-up or not analyzable at the end of the study, we fixed the minimal number of patients per group at 54.

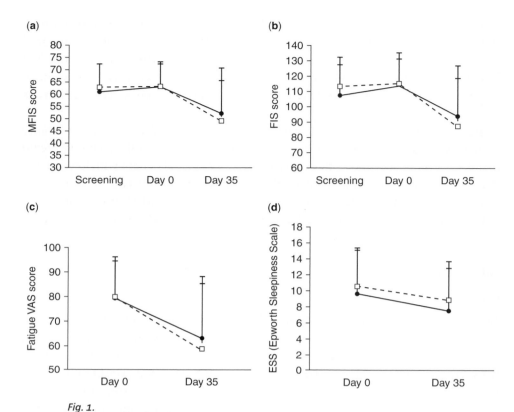

Fig. 1.

Evolution of clinical parameters during the study.

Fatigue was evaluated by the Modified Fatigue Impact Scale (MFIS, **a**), the Fatigue Impact Scale (FIS, **b**) and a Visual Analogic Scale (VAS, **c**). There was a marked improvement of fatigue between day 0 and day 35 in both group, but no difference between groups. Note that the fatigue scores were stable between screening and baseline. Sleepiness was evaluated by the Epworth Sleepiness Scale (ESS, **d**): the improvement of sleepiness was not different between groups. Source: Stankoff *et al.*, 2005.

Trial Methods

This was a randomized, double-blind, parallel group, placebo-controlled study. Screening took place one to four weeks prior to randomization and initiation of therapy. The centralized randomization was then carried out by the study sponsor balancing the treatment assignment by blocks of four within each center. Randomization was stratified according to the EDSS (group 1: EDSS 0–3 inclusive; group 2: EDSS 3.5–6.5 inclusive). The first dispensation of study medication was provided on the same day as randomization.

Titration was as follow: the initial dose was 100 mg twice a day (verum or placebo) and was adjusted depending on the efficacy and safety, by increasing the dose by 100 mg every week, during the first 3 weeks. The maximum dose was 400 mg/day. To adapt the dosage, physicians assessed safety and efficacy using a Visual Analogue

Scale (VAS) by phone once a week. The patients subsequently remained at the same daily dose from day 21 to day 35 (end-of-study).

Primary and Secondary Outcomes

The main outcome variable was a French version of the global MFIS (21 items; score range 0–84, with lower scores indicating less fatigue). MFIS as well as the global FIS were performed at screening, baseline and day 35.

In addition patients completed the Epworth Sleepiness Scale (ESS), a fatigue VAS, the MADRS and the CAS at baseline and at day 35.

Neurological disability was measured using the EDSS score and cognition using the Trail Making Test (part A and part B which reflect the psychomotor speed and mental flexibility, respectively).

Analysis

The primary analysis was conducted on the intent-to-treat (ITT) cohort: all of the patients randomized who took at least one dose of the study medication were included in this population. A secondary analysis was conducted on a per-protocol cohort (PP).

The primary analysis of the global MFIS scores was carried out using a repeated measures analysis of variance: the model was to integrate the measurements taken during screening, baseline and end-of-study visits. The same analysis was performed for the comparison of the FIS and MFIS scores and subscores as well as for ESS, MADRS, and CAS scores. The analysis of the improvement in fatigue on the VAS scale was conducted using a χ^2-test.

Results (Stankoff *et al.*, 2005)

Efficacy

In the modafinil group, the mean global MFIS score was 61 ± 11.4 at selection, 63.1 ± 9.3 at day 0 and improved to 52.3 ± 18.5 at day 35. In the placebo group, the mean MFIS score was 62.9 ± 9.4 at selection, 63.3 ± 10 at day 0 and improved to 49.2 ± 16.6 at day 35. The primary analysis of the global MFIS score did not highlight any significant treatment effect (repeated measures analysis of variance; treatment effect $p = 0.266$). The MFIS scores remained stable between selection and day 0 and decreased during the treatment period, suggesting an improvement of fatigue in both group, with no difference between the two groups. This was confirmed by the comparison of the mean MFIS global scores between baseline and day 35 within each group (analysis of variance for repeated measures), which showed that the difference was highly significant for both the modafinil ($p < 0.001$) and the placebo group ($p < 0.001$). The proportion of patients who experienced an improvement of more than 15 points for the global MFIS score between baseline and day 35 was 35.6% in the modafinil group and 42.8% in the placebo group. Results obtained with the primary criteria were influenced neither by the EDSS stratification, nor by the immunomodulating therapy. They were unchanged with the PP analysis.

The evolution of the global FIS scores were the same as the evolution of MFIS scores: whereas the scores remained stable between screening and day 0, there was an improvement during the treatment period in both groups without any significant drug-placebo differences (ITT analysis: $p = 0.167$).

The ESS scores which measures daytime sleepiness were rather high at baseline in both group: 9.7 ± 5.4 for the modafinil group, 10.6 ± 4.8 for the placebo group. There was a slight improvement of these scores at day 35 whatever the treatment taken, but without a difference between the groups. Similarly, there was an improvement of the fatigue VAS between baseline and day 35, with no significant difference between the groups.

Analysis of parts A and B of the Trail-Making Test, did not show any difference between the two groups.

The change in VAS during the titration period was also evaluated: all patients received 200 mg/day of modafinil or placebo during the first week of treatment and the VAS were captured in all patients at day 7. At this regimen both groups improved compared to baseline, but there was no significant difference between groups. There was no more benefit of modafinil over placebo at day 14 or 21. This suggests that even at lower doses, modafinil was not superior to placebo in this study.

Tolerability

In all, 62 patients (44.9%) presented with at least one adverse event (AE), 34 patients in the modafinil group and 28 patients in the placebo group. The most common AEs concerned nervous, gastrointestinal or psychiatric systems. Only gastrointestinal disorders were significantly more frequent in the modafinil group, but among nervous AEs, insomnia was more frequent in the modafinil group (eight cases in this group compared to only one in the placebo group). Among other sleep disorders, four patients noticed difficulties in falling asleep in each group, and one patient had excessive daytime sleepiness in the modafinil group. The majority of the AEs occurred for a dosage of 200 mg of the study medication (half of AEs in the modafinil group, one third in the placebo group).

There was no modification in neurological disability or in the patient mood status during the study.

Safety

There was no safety concern in this trial.

Unique Aspects of Trial

In previous pilot trials a beneficial effect of modafinil for the treatment of fatigue was suggested (Rammohan *et al.*, 2002; Zifko *et al.*, 2002). However, the lack of randomization as well as the absence of double-blinding in those studies did not allow separation of the placebo-linked and the modafinil-linked benefits, and we speculate that a significant part of the reported improvement was related to a placebo-effect similar to the one that we observed. Our study is the first assessing the efficacy of modafinil for fatigue in MS that meet all standards required for therapeutic evaluation, such as being placebo-controlled, unbiased double blinded, and randomized.

The magnitude of the placebo effect captured in our study is impressive: such a placebo effect, although of smaller magnitude, was observed in previous studies evaluating the efficacy of amantadine or pemoline in MS (Krupp *et al.*,1995). This emphasizes that fatigue is a very subjective symptom, which may be deeply influenced by environment, interaction with physicians and placebo effects. Therefore, whatever the efficacy criteria used in future trial, methods of limiting the placebo effect will be required such as having a placebo wash-in period, as has been used in headache treatment trials (Mathew *et al.*, 1995), or using a longer treatment monitoring period allowing reduction of the placebo effect with time.

Conclusions

Our results show that modafinil was not superior to placebo for the treatment of fatigue in MS, when the whole population of patients complaining of fatigue was considered.

Influence on the Field

Other Recent Advances

Few molecules have been proven to be useful for fatigue in MS. Amantadine has been studied most extensively and appears to improve about one third of patients. Efficacy of pemoline is still a matter of debate, and hepatic toxicity strongly impedes its use in current practice. Potassium channel blockers and SRIs have to be further studied to determine their efficacy in fatigue. Recently a benefit with 1300 mg aspirin per day was suggested in a small cross-over study; this must be confirmed in a larger and more convincing trial (Wingerchuk *et al.*, 2005). Alternative therapies such as acetyl L-carnitine 1 g twice daily (Tomassini *et al.*, 2004), yoga or exercise (Oken, 2004) have been reported to improve fatigue in at least one randomized trial.

How the Trial Results Fit into the Emerging Treatment and Research Framework

We do not conclude that these negative results mean that modafinil has no potential use in MS. The pharmacodynamic properties of this drug mainly relate to the enhancement of wakefulness: therefore further research will have to focus on symptoms related to wakefulness, such as daytime sleepiness or hypersomnia. In many cases these latter complaints may be confounded with fatigue in MS, and interestingly, we found that a significant proportion of our patients also experienced excessive daytime sleepiness as measured with the ESS (ESS, 58/115 patients had a score of 10 or more). Accordingly, preliminary *post hoc* results suggest that among patients complaining of sleepiness, modafinil could provide more benefit than placebo on the physical component of fatigue. Therefore exploring how sleepiness and/or sleep disorders could interfere with the perception of fatigue now represents a promising avenue of research.

In the future it will be crucial to improve our understanding of the pathophysiology of fatigue and related symptoms to introduce some rationale in our therapeutic intervention. Identifying a subgroup of patients with sleepiness or sleep disorders might help to identify the patients that could be improved by modafinil. On the contrary, in the cases where fatigue corresponds to other mechanisms, such as motor weakness, or diffuse neuronal loss, we will have to consider other strategies, for instance motor rehabilitation, exercise, or neuroprotective drugs.

Translation to Clinical Practice

Modafinil should not be used as a first line therapy for fatigue in MS. For patients also complaining of excessive daytime sleepiness, it may represent an alternative that remains to be further investigated.

References

Banerjee, D., Vitiello, M.V., & Grunstein, R.R. (2004). Pharmacotherapy for excessive daytime sleepiness. *Sleep Medicine Reviews*, 8(5), 339–354.

Bever, Jr., C.T., Young, D., Anderson, P.A., Krumholz, A., Conway, K., Leslie, J., *et al.* (1994). The effects of 4-aminopyridine in multiple sclerosis patients: results of a randomized, placebo-controlled, double-blind, concentration-controlled, crossover trial. *Neurology*, 44(6), 1054–1059.

Bever, Jr., C.T., Anderson, P.A., Leslie, J., Panitch, H.S., Dhib-Jalbut, S., Khan, O.A., *et al.* (1996). Treatment with oral 3,4-diaminopyridine improves leg strength in multiple sclerosis patients: results of a randomized, double-blind, placebo-controlled, crossover trial. *Neurology*, 47(6), 1457–1462.

The Canadian MS Research Group. (1987). A randomized controlled trial of amantadine in fatigue associated with multiple sclerosis. *Canadian Journal of Neurological Sciences*, 14(3), 273–278.

Cohen, R.A., & Fisher, M. (1989). Amantadine treatment of fatigue associated with multiple sclerosis. *Archives of Neurology*, 46(6), 676–680.

Comi, G., Leocani, L., Rossi, P., & Colombo, B. (2001). Physiopathology and treatment of fatigue in multiple sclerosis. *Journal of Neurology*, 248(3), 174–179.

Filippi, M., Rocca, M.A., Colombo, B., Falini, A., Codella, M., Scotti, G., et al. (2002). Functional magnetic resonance imaging correlates of fatigue in multiple sclerosis. *Neuroimage*, 15(3), 559–567.

Fisk, J.D., Pontefract, A., Ritvo, P.G., Archibald, C.J., & Murray, T.J. (1994). The impact of fatigue on patients with multiple sclerosis. *Canadian Journal of Neurological Sciences*, 21(1), 9–14.

Krupp, L.B., Coyle, P.K., Doscher, C., Miller, A., Cross, A.H., Jandorf, L., et al. (1995). Fatigue therapy in multiple sclerosis: results of a double-blind, randomized, parallel trial of amantadine, pemoline, and placebo. *Neurology*, 45(11), 1956–1961.

Lin, J.S., Hou, Y., & Jouvet, M. (1996). Potential brain neuronal targets for amphetamine-, methylphenidate-, and modafinil-induced wakefulness, evidenced by c-fos immunocytochemistry in the cat. *Proceedings of the National Academy of Sciences of the United States of America*, 93(24), 14128–14133.

Mathew, N.T., Saper, J.R., Silberstein, S.D., Rankin, L., Markley, H.G., Solomon, S., et al. (1995). Migraine prophylaxis with divalproex. *Archives of Neurology*, 52(3), 281–286.

Murray, T.J. (1985). Amantadine therapy for fatigue in multiple sclerosis. *Canadian Journal of Neurological Sciences*, 12(3), 251–254.

Oken, B.S., Kishiyama, S., Zajdel, D., Bourdette, D., Carlsen, J., Haas, M., et al. (2004). Randomized controlled trial of yoga and exercise in multiple sclerosis. *Neurology*, 62(11), 2058–2064.

Polman, C.H., Bertelsmann, F.W., van Loenen, A.C., & Koetsier, J.C. (1994a). 4-aminopyridine in the treatment of patients with multiple sclerosis. Long-term efficacy and safety. *Archives of Neurology*, 51(3), 292–296.

Polman, C.H., Bertelsmann, F.W., de Waal, R., van Diemen, H.A., Uitdehaag, B.M., van Loenen, A.C., et al. (1994b). 4-Aminopyridine is superior to 3,4-diaminopyridine in the treatment of patients with multiple sclerosis. *Archives of Neurology*, 51(11), 1136–1139.

Rammohan, K.W., Rosenberg, J.H., Lynn, D.J., Blumenfeld, A.M., Pollak, C.P., & Nagaraja, H.N. (2002). Efficacy and safety of modafinil (Provigil) for the treatment of fatigue in multiple sclerosis: a two centre phase 2 study. *Journal of Neurology Neurosurgery and Psychiatry*, 72(2), 179–183.

Ritvo, P.G., Fisk, J.D., Archibald, C.J., Murray, T.J., & Field, C. (1996). Psychosocial and neurological predictors of mental health in multiple sclerosis patients. *Journal of Clinical Epidemiology*, 49(4), 467–472.

Rossini, P.M., Pasqualetti, P., Pozzilli, C., Grasso, M.G., Millefiorini, E., Graceffa, A., et al. (2001). Fatigue in progressive multiple sclerosis: results of a randomized, double-blind, placebo-controlled, crossover trial of oral 4-aminopyridine. *Multiple Sclerosis*, 7(6), 354–358.

Roelcke, U., Kappos, L., Lechner-Scott, J., Brunnschweiler, H., Huber, S., Ammann, W., et al. (1997). Reduced glucose metabolism in the frontal cortex and basal ganglia of multiple sclerosis patients with fatigue: a 18F-fluorodeoxyglucose positron emission tomography study. *Neurology*, 48(6), 1566–1571.

Scammell, T.E., Estabrooke, I.V., McCarthy, M.T., Chemelli, R.M., Yanagisawa, M., Miller, M.S., et al. (2000). Hypothalamic arousal regions are activated during modafinil-induced wakefulness. *Journal of Neuroscience*, 20(22), 8620–8628.

Schwartz, C.E., Coulthard-Morris, L., & Zeng, Q. (1996). Psychosocial correlates of fatigue in multiple sclerosis. *Archives of Physical Medicine and Rehabilitation*, 77(2), 165–170.

Sheean, G.L., Murray, N.M., Rothwell, J.C., Miller, D.H., & Thompson, A.J. (1998). An open-labelled clinical and electrophysiological study of 3,4-diaminopyridine in the treatment of fatigue in multiple sclerosis. *Brain*, 121, 967–975.

Stankoff, B., Waubant, E., Confavreux, C., Edan, G., Debouverie, M., Rumbach, L., *et al.* (2005). French modafinil study group. Modafinil for fatigue in MS: a randomized placebo-controlled double-blind study. *Neurology*, 64, 1139–1143.

Tomassini, V., Pozzilli, C., Onesti, E., Pasqualetti, P., Marinelli, F., Pisani, A., *et al.* (2004). Comparison of the effects of acetyl L-carnitine and amantadine for the treatment of fatigue in multiple sclerosis: results of a pilot, randomised, double-blind, crossover trial. *Journal of Neurological Sciences*, 218(1–2), 103–108.

Van Diemen, H.A., Polman, C.H., van Dongen, T.M., van Loenen, A.C., Nauta, J.J., Taphoorn, M.J., *et al.* (1992). The effect of 4-aminopyridine on clinical signs in multiple sclerosis: a randomized, placebo-controlled, double-blind, cross-over study. *Annals of Neurology*, 32(2), 123–130.

Weinshenker, B.G., Penman, M., Bass, B., Ebers, G.C., & Rice, G.P. (1992). A double-blind, randomized, crossover trial of pemoline in fatigue associated with multiple sclerosis. *Neurology*, 42(8), 1468–1471.

Wingerchuk, D.M., Benarroch, E.E., O'Brien, P.C., Keegan, B.M., Lucchinetti, C.F., Noseworthy, J.H., *et al.* (2005). A randomized controlled crossover trial of aspirin for fatigue in multiple sclerosis. *Neurology*, 64(7), 1267–1269.

Wisor, J.P., & Eriksson, K.S. (2005). Dopaminergic-adrenergic interactions in the wake promoting mechanism of modafinil. *Neuroscience*, 132(4), 1027–1034.

Zifko, U.A., Rupp, M., Schwarz, S., Zipko, H.T., & Maida, E.M. (2002). Modafinil in treatment of fatigue in multiple sclerosis. Results of an open-label study. *Journal of Neurology*, 249(8), 983–987.

Progress in Neurotherapeutics and Neuropsychopharmacology, 1:1, 37–52 © 2006 Cambridge University Press
DOI: 10.1017/S1748232105000054   Printed in the United Kingdom

Radiotherapy with Concurrent and Adjuvant Temozolomide: A New Standard of Care for Glioblastoma Multiforme

Warren P. Mason

Department of Medicine, Princess Margaret Hospital and the University of Toronto, Toronto, Canada;
Email: Warren.Mason@uhn.on.ca

René O. Mirimanoff

Department of Radiation Oncology, Centre Hospitalier Universitaire Vaudois, Lausanne, Switzerland;
Email: Rene_Olivier.Mirimanoff@chuv.ch

Roger Stupp

Multidisciplinary Oncology Center, Centre Hospitalier Universitaire Vaudois, Lausanne, Switzerland;
Email: Roger.Stupp@chuv.ch

Key words: temozolomide; glioblastoma; clinical trial; neurotherapeutics; radiotherapy; quality of life.

Introduction and Overview

Glioblastoma multiforme is the most common and devastating of all primary brain tumors, with median survival typically in the range of 9–12 months with multi-modality treatment (DeAngelis, 2001; Burger & Scheithauer, 1994). Even with aggressive therapeutic approaches to prevent and manage tumor progression, and intense efforts to develop better treatments, survival for patients with glioblastoma has changed little in 30 years. Most patients experience local tumor progression, and usually succumb within months of recurrence. Standard accepted initial therapy for this disease has been maximal feasible surgical resection followed by conformal fractionated radiotherapy. Although not generally considered a chemosensitive tumor, glioblastoma occasionally responds to chemotherapeutic agents, particularly when these drugs are administered for recurrent disease (Brada *et al.*, 2001; Yung *et al.*, 2000). However, no drugs are predictably active against this disease, and most patients with glioblastoma who receive chemotherapy are

Correspondence should be addressed to: Warren P. Mason, MD, Department of Medicine, Princess Margaret Hospital, 610 University Avenue, Suite 18-717, Toronto, Ontario, M5G 2M9, Canada; Ph: +1 416 946 2277; Fax: +1 416 946 2284; Email: Warren.Mason@uhn.on.ca.

usually treated with alkylating agents, historically nitrosoureas and most recently temozolomide (Lesser & Grossman, 1994).

Efforts to improve survival for patients with glioblastoma have included advances in surgical techniques that enable more complete tumor resection, and more sophisticated ways of delivering radiotherapy to the tumor bed while comparatively sparing normal brain; these technical advances have made treatment safer, but have not had a definitive impact on extending survival. Chemotherapy has also been evaluated as initial treatment with surgery and radiotherapy in an attempt to improve dismal survival statistics for glioblastoma. The choice of potential agents for evaluation in glioblastoma has been limited by concerns surrounding effective drug penetration into the central nervous system (CNS), which is protected by a blood–brain barrier that renders tumors at least partly impervious to most drugs. For this reason, most trials that have evaluated adjuvant chemotherapy for glioblastoma have included nitrosoureas, such as carmustine (BCNU) and lomustine (CCNU), which freely cross the intact blood–brain barrier (Rosenblum *et al.*, 1973). Over the last two decades a number of large randomized phase III trials evaluated the efficacy of nitrosourea-based chemotherapy for newly diagnosed malignant glioma, with generally disappointing results (Medical Research Council Brain Tumor Working Party 2001; Shapiro *et al.*, 1989; Chang *et al.*, 1983; Walker *et al.*, 1980, 1978). In these studies, chemotherapy had no definitive impact on median or long-term survival of glioblastoma. Nonetheless, adjuvant chemotherapy was adopted as part of the initial management of glioblastoma, particularly in the USA. An explanation for this practice hinged on a persistent observation from several phase III trials that some patients with glioblastoma seem to benefit from adjuvant chemotherapy (DeAngelis *et al.*, 1996; Fine *et al.*, 1993). This was also confirmed in a recent meta-analysis based on individual patient data of 12 randomized trials that revealed a small but statistically significant benefit for the use of chemotherapy: a 5% increase in survival at 2 years, from 15% to 20% (Stewart, 2002).

Temozolomide is an orally administered, DNA-methylating agent structurally related to dacarbazine, and developed specifically as a treatment for glioma (Stupp *et al.*, 2001; Newlands *et al.*, 1997, 1992). A number of phase II trials in malignant glioma, including glioblastoma, have demonstrated that temozolomide exposure can favorably impact on progression-free survival at 6-months (PFS_{6mo}) and produce occasional radiographic responses with minimal and easily managed toxicities (Brada *et al.*, 2001; Yung *et al.*, 2000, 1999; Newlands *et al.*, 1996). Consequently, temozolomide has become the most common agent for the management of recurrent malignant glioma (Yung, 2000). Very recently, the European Organization for the Research and Treatment of Cancer (EORTC) in collaboration with the National Cancer Institute of Canada Clinical Trials Group (NCIC CTG) reported a successful phase III trial where the addition of temozolomide chemotherapy concurrently with radiotherapy and for up to six cycles of maintenance treatment thereafter improved survival when compared to radiotherapy alone for patients with newly diagnosed glioblastoma (Stupp *et al.*, 2005). This landmark trial is the first study to demonstrate not only a statistically significant, but also a clinically meaningful survival advantage when chemotherapy is included as part of the initial treatment for glioblastoma, and has effectively established a new standard of care for this disease.

Purpose of Trial

Temozolomide had been developed as chemotherapeutic agent aiming in particular at treating malignant brain tumors (Newlands *et al.*, 1997). In recurrent glioma, it has shown some, albeit modest antitumor activity against glioblastoma (Brada *et al.*, 2001). A pilot phase II trial of concurrent temozolomide with fractionated radiotherapy, followed by up to six cycles of adjuvant temozolomide for patients with newly diagnosed glioblastoma, was well-tolerated with acceptable toxicity, and suggested promising clinical activity (Stupp *et al.*, 2002). Based on these preliminary results, the EORTC Brain Tumor Group and Radiotherapy Group and the NCIC CTG, initiated a large multicenter, phase III trial randomizing patients with newly diagnosed glioblastoma to radiotherapy alone versus this combined modality regimen to determine whether the addition of temozolomide in this fashion would improve survival (Stupp *et al.*, 2005).

Agent

Relevant Past Clinical Experience, Phase I and II or Preclinical Data

Temozolomide was developed in the 1980s by the UK Cancer Research Campaign. It is structurally related to dacarbazine, and both drugs are converted systemically to the active metabolite 5-(3-methyl) 1-triazen-1-ly-imidazole-4-carboxamide (MTIC), although in the case of temozolomide conversion occurs spontaneously at normal pH without the need of hepatic activation (Newlands *et al.*, 1997). Temozolomide is an oral agent that is rapidly absorbed with excellent penetration into brain and cerebrospinal fluid (CSF) (Ostermann *et al.*, 2004; Newlands *et al.*, 1992). Maximum plasma concentrations occur within 30–90 min after administration, and excretion is believed to be primarily renal, although dose reduction is not required for patients with renal impairment.

MTIC is a reactive DNA-methylating compound, with preferential affinity for the middle guanine residue of GGG sequences (Clark *et al.*, 1995). Resistance to temozolomide involves two DNA-repair mechanisms, O^6-methylguanine methyltransferase (MGMT) and enzymes involved in DNA mismatch repair (Denny *et al.*, 1994).

Standard dosing of temozolomide consists of a 5-day daily schedule of 200 mg/m^2 (150 mg/m^2 for the first cycle for patients who have had prior chemotherapy) every 28 days (Stupp *et al.*, 2001). The toxicity profile of temozolomide is excellent, with thrombocytopenia being the most common toxicity, severe thrombocytopenia occurring in less than 10% of patients. Other significant toxicities include easily managed nausea and vomiting, fatigue and rarely infections (Stupp *et al.*, 2005). (Supplementary Appendix, http://content.nejm.org/cgi/content/full/352/10/987/DC1). A number of alternate dosing schedules have been evaluated in phase I and II trials, including continuous daily dosing at 75 mg/m^2 for 6–7 weeks (Figueroa *et al.*, 2000; Brock *et al.*, 1998). Continuous daily schedules of temozolomide will exhaust the DNA-repair enzyme MGMT, thus depleting the cells of their repair mechanism (Tolcher *et al.*, 2003). Although extended temozolomide dosing schedules are theoretically appealing, allow administration of over twice the standard total dose per month and have manageable toxicities, superiority of any of the dose-dense schedules over the daily ×5 administration has not yet been shown.

Three pivotal large phase II trials of temozolomide for malignant glioma were conducted in patients who had progressed after intial therapy with surgery, radiotherapy with or without adjuvant chemotherapy (Brada *et al.*, 2001; Yung *et al.*, 2000, 1999). These trials, two in recurrent glioblastoma and one in recurrent anaplastic astrocytoma, used the conventional 5-day temozolomide schedule. For the first time, a chemotherapy agent was evaluated in separate trials for anaplastic astrocytoma (World Health Organization (WHO) grade 3) and glioblastoma (WHO grade 4), two distinct entities with a different natural history. These trials were also unique for using an unconventional primary endpoint, namely the percentage of patients being PFS$_{6mo}$. All patients required a minimum Karnofsky performance status of 70, and pathology and MR images were reviewed centrally. In anaplastic astrocytoma objective radiographic responses was seen in 35% of patients, and disease stabilization occurred in an additional 27% of the total 162 patients enrolled (Yung *et al.*, 1999). Six-month progression-free survival was 46%, and 1-year survival was 56%. In contrast the objective response rate for patients with glioblastoma was only 8% with disease stabilization in an additional 53%, translating in a disease control rate of 61% (Brada *et al.*, 2001). A second phase II trial in glioblastoma was conducted, but designed as a randomized phase II trial administering either temozolomide or procarbazine, another oral alkylating agent (Yung, 2000). Although this trial was not powered for formal statistical comparisons, the 6-month progression-free survival for patients randomized to temozolomide was 21% compared to 8% for those randomized to procarbazine. Although overall median survival was 1.5 months longer in the arm randomized to temozolomide, this difference did not reach statistical significance. In the absence of an established standard treatment for recurrent malignant glioma, temozolomide was received market approval in the USA and throughout Europe in 1999 and 2000. The Food and Drug Administration (FDA) approval was initially granted only for anaplastic astrocytoma based on the observed high response rate. Nonetheless, in clinical practice has been replacing nitrosourea-based chemotherapy increasingly.

Interest in evaluating temozolomide as a treatment for newly diagnosed glioblastoma was based on reports of single-agent activity for recurrent disease, and on occasional observations of objective radiographic tumor response when used as neoadjuvant therapy for glioblastoma before irradiation (Gilbert *et al.*, 2000; Friedman *et al.*, 1998). Furthermore, *in vitro* evidence of temozolomide synergy with radiotherapy, and the potential of circumventing cellular resistance to temozolomide by MGMT depletion when temozolomide is administered in a continuous daily schedule, resulted in a phase II trial that investigated the feasibility of temozolomide administered concomitantly with irradiation and adjuvantly thereafter for 6 months for newly diagnosed glioblastoma (Stupp *et al.*, 2002; Wick *et al.*, 2002; von Rijn *et al.*, 2000; Wedge *et al.*, 1997). In a pilot trial on 64 patients this regimen was found to be safe and well-tolerated with promising efficacy. A median survival of 16 months was reported and 1- and 2-year survival rates of 58% and 31%, respectively. This phase II trial served as the impetus for the EORTC and NCIC CTG phase III study that is the focus of this article (Stupp *et al.*, 2005).

Clinical Trial

Subjects

Patients with newly diagnosed glioblastoma (WHO grade 4 astrocytoma) between the ages of 18 and 70 years of age were eligible to enroll in this trial. Subjects had to have a WHO performance status of 2 or less, and adequate hematologic, renal and hepatic function. Patients had to be on a stable or decreasing dose of corticosteroids for at least 14 days prior to randomization, and had to provide written informed consent to participate.

Between August 2000 and March 2002, 573 patients from 85 institutions in 15 countries were enrolled, and randomized to radiotherapy alone (286 patients) or radiotherapy plus temozolomide (287 patients). The baseline characteristics of patients in both groups were similar, and are summarized in Table 1. The median age of all patients was 56 years, and 84% had debulking surgery. Slightly more patients randomized to radiotherapy alone were receiving corticosteroids at the time of randomization. Central pathology review confirmed the diagnosis of glioblastoma in 93% of patients, 3% had anaplastic gliomas, and in 1% the submitted tumor specimen was insufficient for a reliable diagnosis and in 3% the diagnosis was a non-glial tumor.

Table 1. **Demographic Characteristics of the Patients at Baseline**

CHARACTERISTIC	RADIOTHERAPY (N = 286)	RADIOTHERAPY PLUS TEMOZOLOMIDE (N = 287)
Age (years)		
Median	57	56
Range	23–71	19–70
Age no (%)[a]		
<50 years	81 (28)	90 (31)
≥50 years	205 (72)	197 (69)
Sex no (%)		
Male	175 (61)	185 (64)
Female	111 (39)	102 (36)
WHO performance status no (%)[a,b]		
0	110 (38)	113 (39)
1	141 (49)	136 (47)
2	35 (12)	38(13)
Extent of surgery no (%)[a]		
Biopsy	45 (16)	48 (17)
Debulking	241 (84)	239 (83)
Complete resection	113 (40)	113(39)
Partial resection	128 (45)	126(44)
Time from diagnosis to radiotherapy (week)		
Median	5	5
Range	2.0–12.9	1.7–10.7
Baseline MMSE score no (%)[c]		
30	91 (32)	100 (35)
27–29	97 (34)	96 (33)
≤26	86 (30)	81 (28)
Data missing	12 (4)	10 (3)
Corticosteroid therapy no (%)		
Yes	215 (75)	193 (67)
No	70 (24)	94 (33)
Data missing	1 (<1)	0
Slides available for pathologic review no (%)	246 (86)	239 (83)
Findings on pathologic review no (%)		
Glioblastoma	229 (93)	221 (92)
Anaplastic astrocytoma[d]	9 (4)	7 (3)
Inconclusive material	3 (1)	3 (1)
Others	5 (2)	8 (3)

[a] This characteristic was used as a stratification factor at the time of randomization.
[b] A performance status of 0 denotes asymptomatic, 1 symptomatic and fully ambulatory and 2 symptomatic and in bed less than 50% of the day.
[c] The maximum score on the Mini-Mental State Examination (MMSE) is 30, and scores above 26 are considered to indicate normal mental status.
[d] Anaplastic actrocytoma included oligoastrocytoma.

Trial Methods

Patients had to be randomized to one of two treatment arms within 6 weeks of histologic diagnosis of glioblastoma. Patients were stratified according to age, performance status, extent of resection, and institution. Treatment had to begin within 1 week of randomization.

Radiotherapy was administered as fractionated focal irradiation at a dose of 2 Gy/day, 5 days per week over 6–7 weeks, for a total dose of 60 Gy. Radiotherapy was administered to the postoperative tumor volume plus a 2–3-cm margin. Radiotherapy was planned with dedicated computed tomographic (CT) and three-dimensional planning systems, and delivered by linear accelerators with nominal energy of 6 mV or more. Individual case reviews at selected treatment facilities ensured adequate quality assurance.

Daily temozolomide chemotherapy was administered with radiotherapy at a dose of 75 mg/m^2/day, from the first day of radiotherapy until the last day of radiotherapy, but not for more than 49 days. Following the completion of radiotherapy, patients were given a 4 weeks rest before starting up to six cycles of adjuvant (maintenance) temozolomide chemotherapy administered according to a conventional 5-day schedule every 28 days. Temozolomide was given at a dose of 150 mg/m^2/day for the first cycle, and increased to 200 mg/m^2/day in the absence of severe (WHO grade 3/4) toxicity in the first cycle. *Pneumocystis jiroveci (carinii)* pneumonia prophylaxis with either monthly pentamidine inhalations or trimethoprim-sufometoxazol thrice per week was mandated during concurrent treatment with temozolomide because continuous daily temozolomide frequently induces profound lymphocytopenia. Antiemetic prophylaxis was recommended during daily temozolomide exposure, and mandated during the conventional 5-day treatment.

Instruments/Measures

All patients had baseline bloodwork and CT or MR imaging, physical examination including Mini-Mental State Examination (MMSE) and completed a quality-of-life questionnaire (EORTC QLQ-30 + BCM20); 21–28 days following completion or radiotherapy, and every 3 months thereafter patients underwent complete physical examinations with MMSE and quality-of-life evaluation and radiologic evaluation. Assessment of tumor response was made according to modified WHO criteria, and toxicities were graded according to the National Cancer Institute Common Toxicity Criteria, version 2.0.

Primary and Secondary Outcomes

The primary endpoint was overall survival. Secondary endpoints were progression-free survival, safety, and quality of life.

Analysis

Overall and progression-free survivals were determined by the method of Kaplan and Meier, using two-sided log-rank statistics. The study had an 80% power at a significance level of 0.05 to detect a 33% increase (hazard ration <0.75) in median survival. Analyses were made on an intent-to-treat basis, and the Cox-proportional-hazards method was used to adjust for stratification and confounding factors. Toxicities were reported for the radiotherapy phase (from day 1 of radiotherapy to 28 days after last day of radiotherapy) and adjuvant phase (day 1 of adjuvant chemotherapy until 35 days after last adjuvant cycle) separately.

Results

EFFICACY

The outcome of this trial was analyzed at a median follow-up time of 28 months, by that time 480 patients (84%) had died. The unadjusted hazard ratio for patients randomized to radiotherapy and temozolomide was 0.63 (95% confidence interval (CI), 0.52–0.75, $p < 0.001$). Median overall survival was prolonged by 2.5 months, being 14.6 months in the combined treatment group (95% CI, 13.2–16.8 months) versus 12.1 months (95% CI, 11.2–13.0 months) for those who received radiotherapy alone (Figure 1). The 2-year survival rate was 26.5% (95% CI, 21.2–31.7%) in the experimental arm compared to 10.4% (95% CI, 6.8–14.1%) in the control group. Median progression-free survivals were 6.9 months (95% CI, 5.8–8.2 months) and 5.0 months (95% CI, 4.2–5.5 months), respectively (Figure 2). Clear survival benefit was observed in all patient subgroups, but to a lesser extent in patients with poor performance status (WHO PS 2, $n = 73$ patients) and in those who had biopsy only ($n = 93$ patients).

At study completion, 512 patients (268 in the radiotherapy arm and 244 in the combined treatment arm) had disease progression. In both groups, 23% had a second craniotomy for tumor resection. Seventy-two percent in the radiotherapy alone arm and 58% in the radiotherapy/temozolomide arm received chemotherapy for disease progression. Responses to salvage chemotherapy were not recorded.

TOLERABILITY

The regimen consisting of temozolomide concurrently with radiotherapy and adjuvantly thereafter was generally well-tolerated. In the group randomized to this treatment, 85% completed the concomitant phase of therapy as planned. During the concomitant daily treatment, temozolomide was stopped prematurely in 37 patients (13%), this was due to toxicity in only 12 patients (4%). Adjuvant chemotherapy was administered to 223 patients (78%). Patients who received adjuvant temozolomide received a median of 3 cycles, and 47% completed all six cycles of prescribed therapy. The main reason for failure to start or complete adjuvant chemotherapy was disease progression.

SAFETY

Combined modality treatment with temozolomide and radiotherapy was a safe regimen. Adverse events were analyzed during radiotherapy (with or without concurrent temozolomide), during adjuvant therapy, and for the entire study. No grade 3 or 4 hematologic toxicity was recorded during radiotherapy alone. During concomitant treatment, 7% had grade 3 or 4 hematologic toxicity: 4% had grade 3 or 4 neutropenia, and 3% had grade 3 or 4 thrombocytopenia. During adjuvant

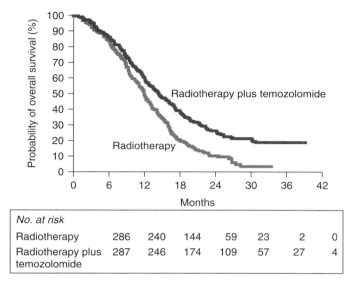

Fig. 1.
Kaplan–Meier estimates of overall survival according to treatment group.
The hazard ratio for death among patients treated with radiotherapy plus temozolomide, as compared with those who received radiotherapy alone, was 0.63 (95% CI, 0.52–0.75; p < 0.001).

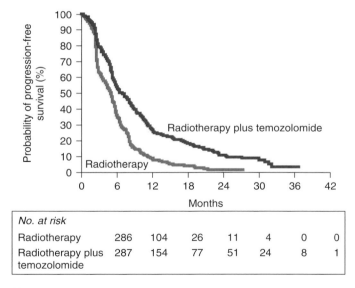

Fig. 2.
Kaplan–Meier estimates of progression-free survival according to treatment group.
The hazard ratio for death or disease progression among patients treated with radiotherapy plus temozolomide, as compared with those treated with radiotherapy alone, was 0.54 (95% CI, 0.45–0.64; p < 0.001).

temozolomide therapy, 14% had grade 3 or 4 myelosuppression: 4% had grade 3 or 4 neutropenia, and 11% had grade 3 or 4 thrombocytopenia.

The most common non-hematologic toxicity was moderate-to-severe fatigue in 26% of the control group, and 33% of those receiving combined treatment. During radiotherapy, severe infections were noted in 2% of patients receiving radiotherapy alone, and 3% receiving radiotherapy plus temozolomide. During the adjuvant phase of treatment, severe infections occurred in 5% of patients. Thromboembolic events occurred in 5%, 16 patients in the radiotherapy group, and 12 patients in the combined treatment group. At a median follow-up of 2 years, no treatment-induced, late toxic effects have been seen, neither cognitive deficits nor hematologic malignancies.

UNIQUE ASPECTS OF TRIAL

Temozolomide is a remarkable chemotherapeutic agent because it possesses several important characteristics that made its evaluation in newly diagnosed glioblastoma appealing: good CNS penetration, excellent toxicity profile even when administered chronically, and phase II data suggesting activity in high-grade glioma. The most compelling aspect of this trial was the continuous daily administration of this agent during radiotherapy. Whether the efficacy of this regimen is a result of concomitant temozolomide administration causing therapeutic synergy with irradiation, depletion of MGMT, or benefit from early and continuous chemotherapy is unknown. Moreover, whether adjuvant or maintenance chemotherapy with temozolomide also contributed to favorable outcome is unclear; previous experience with adjuvant chemotherapy for glioblastoma has been uniformly disappointing.

Of note is that the majority of patients randomized to initially radiotherapy alone received temozolomide salvage therapy at progression. Despite this crossover, the patient receiving temzolomide as part of an initial combined modality therapy fared much better than sparing the chemotherapy for the recurrent situation.

CONCLUSIONS

The administration of temozolomide concurrently with radiotherapy and for up to 6 cycles thereafter for newly diagnosed glioblastoma represents the first clinically meaningful advance in the treatment of this disease in over three decades, and should be considered the new standard of care for most patients with this cancer.

Influence on the Field

Other Recent Advances

A recent study by Hegi *et al.* using tumor specimens of patients enrolled in the EORTC and NCIC CTG trial of temozolomide with radiotherapy for newly diagnosed glioblastoma has linked temozolomide resistance to tumor *MGMT* promoter methylation status (Hegi *et al.*, 2005). MGMT is a DNA-repair protein that is believed responsible for the resistance of gliomas to alkylating agents such as nitrosoureas and temozolomide. Epigenetic silencing of the *MGMT* gene by promoter hypermethylation reduces *MGMT* gene expression; for unknown reasons, hypermethylation of the *MGMT* promoter is present in approximately half of the glioblastoma (Esteller *et al.*, 1999). Previous retrospective studies have associated *MGMT* promoter methylation with prolonged survival in patients with glioblastoma who receive radiotherapy and alkylating chemotherapy (Hegi *et al.*, 2004; Esteller *et al.*, 2000; Jaeckle *et al.*, 1998).

Hegi *et al.* evaluated *MGMT* promoter methylation status of tumor specimens from 307 of 573 patients enrolled in the EORTC and NCIC CTG trial. A two-step PCR-based methodology was used to determine promoter methylation status. Promotor methylation status could be determined in 206 of 307 tumor specimens, and survival analyses were performed on the subset for which methylation status was known. Importantly, the clinical profile and overall survival outcome of this subset was representative of the entire trial cohort of 573 patients. Of the 206 cases, *MGMT* promoter methylation was present in 92 (44.7%) and absent in 114 (55.3%). Promoter methylation was associated with superior overall survival, regardless of whether patients were assigned to temozolomide with radiotherapy or radiotherapy alone at study enrollment (hazard ratio for death 0.45, 95% CI, 0.32–0.61). Independent of treatment assignment, median overall survival for patients with a methylated *MGMT* promoter was 18.2 months (95% CI, 15.5–22.0 months) versus 12.2 months for patients without *MGMT* methylation (95% CI, 11.4–13.5 months). More strikingly, for patients with *MGMT* promoter methylation assigned to combined modality treatment, median survival was 21.7 months (95% CI, 17.4–30.4 months) and 2-year survival was 46% (95% CI, 31.2–60.8%). Patients who had unmethylated *MGMT* promoter assigned to combined modality treatment had a median survival of only 12.7 months (95% CI, 11.6–14.4 months) and a 2-year survival of only 13.8% (95% CI, 4.8–22.7%). This difference, which was statistically significant, indicates that *MGMT* promoter methylation status is an important predictor of survival benefit from combined temozolomide and radiotherapy for glioblastoma. Furthermore, a multivariate analysis using the Cox-proportional-hazards model identified *MGMT* promoter methylation status as the most significant independent prognostic factor for survival ($p < 0.001$). Thus, *MGMT* promoter methylation status emerges as the first molecular genetic determinant of outcome and treatment response for glioblastoma.

How the Trial Results Fit into the Emerging Treatment and Research Framework

The use of concurrent and adjuvant temozolomide with radiotherapy for patients with newly diagnosed glioblastoma has become the new standard of care for patients with this disease (DeAngelis, 2005). However, improvement of median survival is modest, and patients without *MGMT* promoter hypermethylation and thus a functional repair enzyme derive little if any benefit from this new combined modality treatment. Strategies to overcome MGMT-mediated temozolomide resistance include those that increase exposure of temozolomide by prolonging the duration of conventional adjuvant therapy or by increasing the intensity of temozolomide therapy by continuous "daily" adjuvant therapy. Such a trial is currently under development by the Radiation Therapy Oncology Group (RTOG) in collaboration with the EORTC (RTOG0525/EORTC26052). This study will include *MGMT* promoter methylation status as a stratification factor as a means of confirming prospectively the prognostic and predictive significance of this molecular marker for glioblastoma. This requires that sufficient and adequate tissue is available on all patients.

Patients older than age 70 were excluded from the EORTC/NCIC trial, leaving the role of temozolomide in the management of glioblastoma in the elderly uncertain (Chinot *et al.*, 2004; Brandes *et al.*, 2003). Although survival of elderly patients with glioblastoma is poor, and therapy in this age group may induce serious toxicities and a detrimental impact on quality of life, clinical trials evaluating temozolomide for newly diagnosed glioblastoma in the elderly are needed to guide clinical management.

There is currently no proven role for chemotherapy in the initial management of anaplastic astrocytoma and anaplastic oligodendroglioma despite evidence that such tumors with 1p and 19q loss of heterozygosity are remarkably chemosensitive neoplasms (van den Bent *et al.*, 2003; Ino *et al.*, 2001; Cairncross *et al.*, 1998). Recently reported large randomized phase III trials evaluating PCV chemotherapy for newly diagnosed anaplastic oligodendroglial tumors have failed to show a survival benefit for adjuvant chemotherapy (van den Bent *et al.*, 2005; Cairncross *et al.*, 2004). Despite these negative outcomes, trials that evaluate temozolomide chemotherapy, including its combination with radiotherapy, for newly diagnosed anaplastic gliomas are needed.

Relevant FDA Issues

Based on the EORTC/NCIC CTG phase III trial, the FDA of the United States approved temozolomide for first-line treatment of glioblastoma on 15 March 2005. Specifically, temozolomide has been approved in combination with focal radiotherapy (concomitant phase) followed by up to six cycles of temozolomide monotherapy for adults with newly diagnosed glioblastoma. The FDA has mandated *Pneumocystis carinii* prophylaxis during the concomitant phase, and has issued a warning that temozolomide like all alkylating agents may be associated with an increased risk for developing myelodysplastic syndromes and acute leukemias.

Translation into Clinical Practice

Influence on Clinical Guidelines

Concomitant and adjuvant temozolomide with radiotherapy is rapidly becoming the new standard of care for most patients with newly diagnosed glioblastoma. In addition to FDA approval, this regimen has been approved by the 25 European Union member states. It is anticipated that this new indication will be approved for temozolomide wherever the drug is marketed.

Treatment Algorithm

A diagnosis of glioblastoma can only be established at the time of surgery, and patients with this disease should have a maximal feasible resection at that time. Subsequently, patients who are to receive radical courses of focal radiotherapy (60 Gy) should also receive concomitant temozolomide. Following the concomitant phase of treatment, all patients should be considered for monthly temozolomide monotherapy, provided they remain candidates for ongoing anticancer therapy. The adjuvant phase of temozolomide therapy has been evaluated and approved for only six cycles. Although continuing temozolomide chemotherapy for 1 year and beyond is usually safe, there is currently no evidence that prolonged treatment translates in improved outcome. In patients demonstrating continued radiographic response after 6 cycles, consideration of prolonged treatment may be justified.

Summary of How to Treat the Disorder Incorporating the Results of the New Trial Data

Concurrent and adjuvant temozolomide with radiotherapy is the new standard of care for patients with newly diagnosed glioblastoma following maximal surgical resection. Most patients with this disease should receive this regimen, exceptions being those with very poor performance status, and the very elderly. Although *MGMT* promoter methylation status appears to be a predictive factor for good outcome following this regimen, results are preliminary and this test should not be used clinically to guide management decisions at this time. Although the duration of the adjuvant phase of temozolomide chemotherapy remains controversial, treatment should not continue indefinitely until progression, particularly if disease stabilization has been present for several months. Rather, to help answer these questions, patients with newly diagnosed glioblastoma should be encouraged to consider enrollment into the RTOG and EORTC sponsored trial to evaluate prospectively the significance of *MGMT* promoter methylation status, and a more dose intense temozolomide regimen. Alternative strategies build on adding a targeted agent (e.g. EGFR inhibitors, VEGF inhibitors or integrin inhibitors targeting neoangiogenesis) on the backbone of this newly developed regimen. For patients who have disease progression during or shortly after the adjuvant phase of treatment, enrollment in a clinical trial should be considered. For those who experience late progression (at least 6 months following last temozolomide exposure), retreatment with temozolomide remains an option. Ultimately, however, further advances in the management of this disease will require discovery of new active agents, and patients should be encouraged to participate in trials that explore novel therapeutics.

References

Brada, M., Hoang-Xuang, K., Rampling, R., *et al.* (2001). Multicenter phase II trial of temozolomide in patients with glioblastoma multiforme at first relapse. *Annals of Oncology*, 12, 259–266.

Brandes, A., Vastola, F., Basso, U., *et al.* (2003). A prospective study on glioblastoma in the elderly. *Cancer*, 97, 657–662.

Brock, C., Newlands, E., Wedge, S., *et al.* (1998). Phase I trial of temozolomide using an extended continuous oral schedule. *Cancer Research*, 58, 4363–4367.

Burger, P., & Scheithauer, B. (1994). *Tumors of the Central Nervous System*, Washington, D.C: Armed Forces Institute of Pathology.

Cairncross, J.G., Ueki, K., Zlatescu, M.C., *et al.* (1998). Specific genetic predictors of chemotherapeutic response and survival in patients with anaplastic oligodendrogliomas. *Journal of National Cancer Institute*, 90, 1473–1479.

Cairncross, J.G., Seiferheld, W., Shaw, E., *et al.* (2004). An intergroup randomized controlled clinical trial (RTC) of chemotherapy plus radiation (RT) versus RT alone for pure and mixed anaplastic oligodendrogliomas: Initial report of RTOG 94-02. *Journal of Clinical Oncology*, 22 (July 15 Suppl.), 1500.

Chang, C., Horton, J., Schoenfeld, D., *et al.* (1983). Comparison of postoperative radiotherapy and combined postoperative radiotherapy and chemotherapy in the multidisciplinary management of malignant gliomas. *Cancer*, 52, 997–1007.

Chinot, O.L., Barrie, M., Frauger, E., *et al.* (2004). Phase II study of temozolomide without radiotherapy in newly diagnosed glioblastoma multiforme in an elderly populations. *Cancer*, 100, 2208–2214.

Clark, A., Deans, B., Stevens, M., *et al.* (1995). Anti-tumor imidazotetrazines: synthesis of novel imidazotetrazines and related bicyclic heterocycles to probe the mode of action of the antitumor drug temozolomide. *Journal of Medicinal Chemistry*, 38, 1493–1504.

DeAngelis, L.M. (2001). Brain tumors. *New England Journal of Medicine*, 344, 114–123.

DeAngelis, L.M. (2005). Chemotherapy for brain tumors – a new beginning. *New England Journal of Medicine*, 352, 1036–1038.

DeAngelis, L.M., Burger, P., Green, S., *et al.* (1996). Adjuvant chemotherapy for malignant glioma: Who benefits? *Annals of Neurology*, 40, 491–492.

Denny, B., Wheelhouse, R., Stevens, M., *et al.* (1994). NMR and molecular modeling investigation of the mechanism of activation of the antitumor drug temozolomide and its interaction with DNA. *Biochemistry*, 33, 9045–9051.

Esteller, M., Hamilton, S., Burger, P., Baylin, S., & Herman, J. (1999). Inactivation of the DNA repair gene O6-methylguanine-DNA methyltransferase by promotor hypermethylation is a common event in primary human neoplasia. *Cancer Research*, 59, 793–797.

Esteller, M., Garcia-Foncillas, J., Andion, E., *et al.* (2000). Inactivation of the DNA-repair gene MGMT and the clinical response of gliomas to alkylating agents. *New England Journal of Medicine*, 343, 1350–1354.

Figueroa, J., Tolcher, A., Denis, L., *et al.* (2000). Protracted cyclic administration of temozolomide is feasible: a phase I and pharmacokinetic-pharmacodynamic study. *Proceedings of American Society Clinical Oncology*, 19, 22a [Abstract 868].

Fine, H.A., Dear, K.B.J., Loeffler, J.S., *et al.* (1993). Meta-analysis of radiation therapy with and without adjuvant chemotherapy for malignant gliomas in adults. *Cancer*, 71, 2585–2597.

Friedman, H., McLendon, R., Kerby, T., *et al.* (1998). DNA mismatch repair and O6-alkylguanine-DNA alkyltransferase analysis and response to Temodal in newly diagnosed malignant glioma. *Journal of Clinical Oncology*, 16, 3851–3857.

Gilbert, M., Olson, J., Yung, W.K.A., *et al.* (2000). Preirradiation treatment of newly diagnosed anaplastic astrocytomas and glioblastoma multiforme using temozolomide. *Neuro-Oncology*, 2, 264 [Abstract 77].

Lesser, G.J., & Grossman, S. (1994). The chemotherapy of high-grade astrocytomas. *Seminars in Oncology*, 21, 220–235.

Hegi, M.E., Diserens, A.-C., Godard, S., *et al.* (2004). Clinical trial substantiates the predictive value of O-6-methylguanine-DNA methyltransferase promotor methylation in glioblastoma patients treated with temozolomide. *Clinical Cancer Research*, 10, 1871–1874.

Hegi, M.E., Diserens, A.-C., Gorlia, T., *et al.* (2005). MGMT gene silencing and benefit from temozolomide in glioblastoma. *New England Journal of Medicine*, 352, 997–1003.

Ino, Y., Betensky, R., Zlatescu, M., *et al.* (2001). Molecular subtypes of anaplastic oligodendroglioma: implications for patient management at diagnosis. *Clinical Cancer Research*, 7, 839–845.

Jaeckle, K., Eyre, H., Townsend, J., *et al.* (1998). Correlation of tumor O6 methylguanine-DNA methyltransferase levels with survival of malignant astrocytoma patients treated with bis-chloroethylnitrosourea: a Southwest Oncology Group study. *Journal of Clinical Oncology*, 16, 3310–3315.

Medical Research Council Brain Tumor Working Party. (2001). Randomized Trial of Procarbazine, Lomustine, and Vincristine in the Adjuvant Treatment of High-Grade Astrocytoma: A Medical research Council Trial. *Journal of Clinical Oncology*, 19, 509–518.

Newlands, E., Blackledge, G., Slack, J., *et al.* (1992). Phase I trial of temozolomide (CCRG 81045: M and B 39831: NSC 362856). *British Journal of Cancer*, 65, 287–291.

Newlands, E.S., Blackledge, G.R.P., Slack, J.A., *et al.* (1996). The Charing Cross Hospital experience with temozolomide in patients with gliomas. *European Journal of Cancer*, 32A, 2236–2241.

Newlands, E., Stevens, M., Wedge, S., Wheelhouse, R., & Brock, C. (1997). Temozolomide: a review of its discovery, chemical properties, pre-clinical development and clinical trials. *Cancer Treatment Reviews*, 23, 35–61.

Ostermann, S., Csajka, C., Buclin, T., *et al.* (2004). Plasma and cerebrospinal fluid population pharmacokinetics of temozolomide in malignant glioma patients. *Clinical Cancer Research*, 10, 3728–3736.

Rosenblum, M.L., Reynolds, J.A.F., Smith, K.A., *et al.* (1973). Chloroethyl-cyclohexyl-nitrosourea (CCNU) in the treatment of malignant brain tumors. *Journal of Neurosurgery*, 39, 306–314.

Shapiro, W., Green, S., Burger, P., *et al.* (1989). Randomized trial of three chemotherapy regimens and two radiotherapy regimens in postoperative treatment of malignant glioma. *Journal of Neurosurgery*, 71, 1–9.

Stewart, L. (2002). Chemotherapy in adult high-grade glioma: a systematic review and meta-analysis of individual patient data from 12 randomized trials. *Lancet*, 359, 1011–1018.

Stupp, R., Gander, M., Leyvraz, S., & Newlands, E. (2001). Current and future developments in the use of temozolomide for the treatment of brain tumors. *Lancet Oncology*, 2, 552–560.

Stupp, R., Dietrich, P.-Y., Kralijevic, S.O., *et al.* (2002). Promising survival for patients with newly diagnosed glioblastoma multiforme treated with concomitant radiation plus temozolomide followed by adjuvant temozolomide. *Journal of Clinical Oncology*, 20, 1375–1382.

Stupp, R., Mason, W.P., van den Bent, M.J., *et al.* (2005). Radiotherapy plus concomitant and adjuvant temozolomide for newly diagnosed glioblastoma. *New England Journal of Medicine*, 352, 987–996.

Tolcher, A., Gerson, S., Denis, L., *et al.* (2003). Marked inactivation of O6-alkylguanine-DNA alkyltransferase activity with protracted temozolomide schedules. *British Journal of Cancer*, 88, 1004–1011.

van den Bent, M.J., Chinot, O.-L., & Cairncross, J.G. (2003). Recent developments in the molecular characterization and treatment of oligodendroglial tumors. *Neuro-Oncology*, 5, 128–138.

van den Bent, M.J., Delattre, J.-Y., Brandes, A., *et al.* (2005). First analysis of EORTC trial 26951, a randomized phase III study of adjuvant PCV chemotherapy in patients with highly anaplastic oligodendroglioma. *Proceedings of American Society Clinical Oncology*, 23, 115s [Abstract 1503].

von Rijn, J., Heimans, J., van den Berg, J., van den Valk, P., & Slotman, B. (2000). Survival of human glioma cells treated with various combinations of temozolomide and X-rays. *International Journal of Radiation Oncology Biology Physics*, 47, 779–784.

Walker, M., Alexander, E., Hunt, W., *et al.* (1978). Evaluation of BCNU and/or radiotherapy in the treatment of anaplastic gliomas. *Jounal of Neurosurgery*, 49, 333–343.

Walker, M., Green, S., Byar, D., *et al.* (1980). Randomized comparison of radiotherapy and nitrosoureas for the treatment of malignant glioma after surgery. *New England Journal of Medicine*, 303, 1323–1329.

Wedge, S., Porteous, J., Glaser, M., Marcus, K., & Newlands, E. (1997). *In vitro* evaluation of temozolomide combined with X-irradiation. *Anticancer Drugs*, 8, 92–97.

Wick, W., Wick, A., Schulz, J.B., *et al.* (2002). Prevention of irradiation-induced glioma cell invasion by temozolomide involves caspase 3 activity and cleavage of focal adhesion kinase. *Cancer Research*, 62, 1915–1919.

Yung, W.K.A. (2000). Temozolomide in malignant glioma. *Seminars in Oncology*, 27, 27–34.

Yung, W.K.A., Prados, M.D., Yaya-Tur, P., *et al.* (1999). Multicenter phase II trial of temozolomide in patients with anaplastic astrocytoma or anaplastic oligoastrocytoma at first relapse. *Journal of Clinical Oncology*, 17, 2762–2771.

Yung, W.K.A., Albright, R.E., Olson, J., *et al.* (2000). A phase II study of temozolomide versus procarbazine in patients with glioblastoma multiforme at first relapse. *British Journal of Cancer*, 85, 588–593.

Progress in Neurotherapeutics and Neuropsychopharmacology, 1:1, 53–61 © 2006 Cambridge University Press
DOI: 10.1017/S1748232105000066   Printed in the United Kingdom

Treating Migraine Attacks ASAP: Concept and Methodological Issues

Natalie J. Wiendels and Michel D. Ferrari

Department of Neurology, Leiden University Medical Centre, Leiden, The Netherlands;
Email: M.D.Ferrari@LUMC.NL

Key words: Migraine; clinical trials; neurotherapeutics; triptans; allodynia; placebo effects; responder rates.

Introduction

Migraine is a common neurovascular disorder characterised by recurrent attacks of moderate to severe headache with nausea and/or photo- and phonophobia. Triptans, selective serotonin $5\text{-HT}_{1B/1D}$ agonists, are specific acute migraine drugs of which efficacy and safety are well established in numerous clinical trials (Goadsby *et al.*, 2002; Ferrari *et al.*, 2001). Efficacy is usually presented as the response rate, the proportion of patients whose headache improved from severe or moderate pain at baseline to mild or no pain at 2-h post-dose (Figure 1) (Tfelt-Hansen *et al.*, 2000). Consequently, in clinical trials of triptans in acute migraine, patients have traditionally been required to take their medication only when their pain had reached a moderate or severe intensity. There are good methodological reasons for this somewhat artificial design. If patients wait until a moderate or severe pain level has been reached, it is more likely that true migraine headaches are being treated rather than a non-migraine (e.g. tension-type) headache (Tfelt-Hansen *et al.*, 2000). Delayed treatment should also minimise the placebo response, allowing for spontaneous resolution of possible short, non-migraine headaches. It also simplifies the assessment of the improvement as all patients start from a similar level of baseline pain rather than from different levels: a shift from severe to moderate pain is not the same as improvement from mild to no pain.

In clinical practice, however, patients obviously prefer to experience pain as little and as briefly as possible. Intuitively, early treatment of migraine attacks when the headache is still mild seems preferable and should result in higher responder

Correspondence should be addressed to: Michel D. Ferrari, MD, PhD, Department of Neurology, Leiden University Medical Centre, Albinusdreef 2, 2333 ZA Leiden, P.O. Box 9600, 2300 RC Leiden, The Netherlands; Ph: +31 71 5262895; Fax: +31 71 5248253; Email: M.D.Ferrari@LUMC.NL.

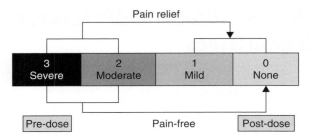

Fig. 1.
Migraine pain intensity is assessed on a 4-point severity scale where 0: no pain, 1: mild, 2: moderate and 3: severe.

rates than when the headache is treated later at moderate or severe intensity. This would obviously be better for the patient but also would enhance the perception of the efficacy of triptans. Clinical researchers and pharmaceutical companies alike are therefore searching for novel trial designs allowing patients to treat early while the headache is still mild, in the hope that this regimen will show better responder rates than those obtained with the traditional trial designs. In this review we will discuss the arguments in favour and against the widely marketed "early treatment" approach. We will also highlights some misconceptions and important pitfalls in the interpretation of the results of trials implementing this design. These issues have been discussed earlier in two articles (Ferrari, 2005, 2004).

Neurobiological Evidence Supporting Early Treatment

There is some neurobiological evidence supporting early triptan treatment. In a series of elegant studies, Burstein and colleagues (2004, 2000) have shown that central sensitisation may occur during the course of migraine attacks, as evidenced by the development of cutaneous allodynia in over 70% of their patients. In animal models they showed that early application of triptans blocks the development of central sensitisation, whereas late application of triptans is insufficient to counteract established central sensitisation. This was confirmed in a small study in 31 patients who treated 34 migraine attacks with allodynia and 27 attacks without allodynia (Burstein *et al.*, 2004). Patients were pain-free 2 h after triptan therapy in 15% of allodynic attacks in comparison with 93% of non-allodynic attacks. Patients who did not develop allodynia were highly likely to achieve freedom from pain after triptan therapy at any time after the onset of pain. They concluded that triptan therapy was more likely to be effective if administered before rather than after the development of cutaneous allodynia and described the process of therapy with triptans as a race against the development of central sensitisation.

Clinical Trial Evidence Favouring Early Treatment

There is a growing number of reports in the scientific literature describing clinical trials that purport to demonstrate the benefits of "early" treatment (Cady *et al.*, 2004, 2000; Dowson *et al.*, 2004; Klapper *et al.*, 2004; Mathew *et al.*, 2004; Scholpp *et al.*, 2004; Mathew, 2003; Pascual & Cabarrocas, 2002). Some of these are retrospective analyses of protocol violators, patients who failed to comply with the trial instructions and accidentally treated mild headache instead of moderate or severe pain. *Post-hoc* analyses in three sumatriptan trials, for example, found that patients who had treated their headache while pain was mild had higher pain-free response rates and lower rates of redosing than those who had treated when their headache pain was moderate to severe (Cady *et al.*, 2000). Two randomised prospective trials that studied the efficacy of early treatment with triptans found high responder rates for improvement to pain-free at 2-h post-dose (Klapper *et al.*, 2004; Scholpp *et al.*, 2004). As these responder rates were higher than historical responder rates obtained in older trials using the traditional design of treating moderate or severe pain, the authors concluded that: (i) their findings extend the results of earlier trials that had been using historical comparisons and (ii) "early treatment", when the pain is still mild, affords improved efficacy over "late treatment" when the pain is moderate or severe.

Methodological and Clinical Pitfalls

Not only does it seem intuitively obvious that treating a migraine attack early in its course is preferable to delaying therapy, there also seems to be neurobiological and clinical evidence to support this approach. But the evidence favouring early treatment must be carefully examined. There are a number of methodological and clinical pitfalls that need to be considered, before accepting the hypothesis that treating early affords clinically relevant improved efficacy without increased risk of medication-overuse headaches.

The Allodynia Dilemma

In Burstein's studies, both allodynia and triptan efficacy were assessed unblinded, without placebo control. This complicates the interpretation of the results. Many placebo-controlled clinical trials with triptans have failed to show a difference in efficacy between patients treated very early, so presumably before allodynia had developed, and patients treated late, so presumably with a high proportion of patients with allodynia (Plosker & McTavish, 1994; The Subcutaneous Sumatriptan International Study Group, 1991). The observation that patients with allodynia may still respond well to subcutaneous triptan treatment was recently confirmed in a study by Diamond & Freitag (2004). In conclusion, the jury is still out whether late treatment and allodynia predict poor response to triptans. An interesting alternative hypothesis could be that the central sensitisation process may increase the risk of recurrence rather than the lack of initial relief.

Historical Comparisons and the Illustrious Placebo Effect

The historical evidence from *post-hoc* analyses can be regarded as hypothesis generating only. Comparisons of response rates in patients treating mild or early headaches in new trials with response rates from old trials in which patients were instructed to treat moderate or severe headaches are not instructive, as they cannot take into account differences in study designs and patient types, or the possible effect of higher placebo rates in patients treating their headache early. The therapeutic gains in comparison with placebo in the current trials of "mild" migraine can be, owing to possibly higher placebo response rates, in fact similar or even smaller than those in the previous trials of "severe" migraine. Just comparing absolute response rates in different study designs, without accounting for different placebo responses, may be misleading. A patient may improve after taking placebo, or indeed medication, for several reasons. It is important to remember that migraine attacks are self-limiting. There might be regression to the mean (i.e. patients may seek medical help or take medication at the peak of severity, and the severity would have declined thereafter irrespective of medication) or the attack might follow a short natural course. The diagnosis may also be incorrect; for example, the patient might treat a tension-type headache attack rather than a true migraine attack, so the patient would be treating a condition with a better outcome. This is even more likely when patients start treating attacks very early on, prior to the development of associated symptoms such as nausea, vomiting, and phono- and photophobia that are important features in discriminating migraine attacks from tension-type headaches. Finally, some patients will experience a true placebo effect, a response that may be mediated by endorphins.

Treating "Early" versus Treating "Mild"

Furthermore, in the past, "treating early" and "treating mild" have been incorrectly used as interchangeable terms. A clinical trial requires a balanced distribution of the baseline characteristics of the study populations, particularly disease severity, duration, and other prognostic factors. This, after all, is the purpose of randomisation. Migraine attacks can progress slowly or rapidly (Figure 2). Although the same level of pain intensity may be reached ultimately in the two types of

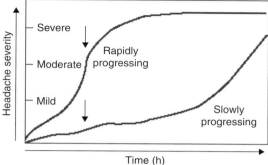

Rapidly versus slowly progressing migraine attacks

Fig. 2.
The two types of migraine, rapidly progressing and slowly progressing. Treating "early" (arrow) may be the same as treating "mild" in a patient with slowly progressing migraine, but early treatment may not equate with treatment of mild pain in an individual with rapidly progressing migraine.

attacks, it will take longer in the slowly progressing type. Treating early may be the same as treating mild pain in a slowly progressing migraine attack, but early treatment may not equate with treatment of mild pain in a rapidly progressing migraine attack (Foley *et al.*, 2005). If early and late treatment are to be compared fairly without considering pain intensity, the comparison needs to be made in one type of attack group only, either in those with slowly progressing attacks (in whom early treatment will equate with treatment of mild pain) or in those with rapidly progressing attacks (in whom treating early does not always mean treating mild pain). In order to minimise this imbalance only one type of patients should be included in a study and asked to treat attacks either early or late, preferentially in a randomised, within-patient, cross-over design. Only in the slowly progressing type, will this equate with "treating mild" versus "treating severe".

Therapeutic Gain versus Comparing Absolute Responder Rates

When asked to treat early, migraine patients may accidentally treat short migraine or tension-type headache attacks. This could result in accidental improvement due to natural course rather than pharmacological mechanisms. Expectation of relief triggered by information in the patient informed consent that early treatment may be superior could bias patients and therefore may promote a placebo *effect*. Thus the effect must be placebo-controlled and the analysis should be based on comparing the *therapeutic gains* of active over placebo treatment for early versus later treatment rather than the absolute rates for *verum*. This could be done in a four-arm parallel-group design, in which patients treat one attack randomly allocated to one of four treatments: (i) early with placebo; (ii) early with *verum*; (iii) late with placebo; or (iv) late with *verum*. Even better, but more complicated, one could use a partial parallel-group/cross-over design, in which patients are randomised to treat two attacks early or two attacks late, one with placebo and one with *verum*. A full cross-over design in which patients treat four attacks would probably be too complicated.

Pain-Free at 2 h is a Misleading Endpoint in Early Treatment Trials

The outcome measure used in a trial of early versus late treatment of migraine raises further issues. Pain-free 2-h post-dose is now recommended as the primary efficacy measure in clinical trials of migraine therapy (using the traditional design) rather than 2-h pain relief, the primary endpoint used in most earlier trials (Tfelt-Hansen *et al.*, 2000). Note that in the traditional design *improvement* from moderate or severe pain down to mild or no pain is being assessed. These measures, however, may not be appropriate for a trial of early treatment in which the aim is to *prevent progression* of pain. The sustained pain-free outcome, that is freedom from pain at 2-h post-dose *without* recurrence of the pain during the subsequent 22 h and without the need for additional medication is a more appropriate endpoint. This endpoint can be used to assess the immediate effect of medication on migraine of any baseline severity and encompasses both improvement and prevention of progression, thus reflecting what patients want from treatment; pain-free as soon as possible and for the duration of the attack. The sustained pain-free endpoint is both clinically relevant and realistic, and patients achieving this outcome measure will have experienced a true blockade of their attack. Treatment success rates in the sustained pain-free parameter will, inevitably, be lower than those in the 2-h pain-free parameter, but this will lessen the potential for unreasonably high expectations to engender dissatisfaction with treatment outcomes.

The Optimal Design for Early Treatment Trials

For an optimal and clinically relevant comparison of early versus later treatment, the following guidelines should be considered:

- Outcome measure: sustained pain-free, that is pain-free by 2-h post-dose and for the subsequent 22 h without use of additional pain medication within that time frame.

- Inclusion: inclusion of only one type of patients, either those with slowly progressing attacks or those with rapidly progressing attacks.

- Design: choice between the following options:
  - For a four-arm parallel-group design, random allocation of the patients to one of four treatments: (i) early with placebo; (ii) early with *verum*; (iii) late with placebo; and (iv) late with *verum*.

– For a two-arm parallel-group design, random allocation of the patients to treating two attacks either early or late: one attack with placebo and one with *verum* in randomised order.
– Statistical analysis should be based on comparing the *therapeutic gains* (*verum* minus placebo) for early versus late treatment rather than comparing absolute rates for *verum*.
– Conclusions apply only to the type of patients included in the trial and cannot be extrapolated to the other type.
– When only patients with slowly progressing attacks have been included, one can assume that the findings may also apply to "treating mild" versus "treating severe".
– For scientific reasons, one may include testing for the presence of allodynia, but by an investigator who is blinded to the clinical status of the patient and the treatment protocol; this will complicate the study considerably.

Risks Associated with Recommending Early Treatment

There is also a danger in advising early medication for all patients as this may increase the risk of medication-overuse headache. Medication-overuse headache is a growing problem worldwide. Epidemiological data suggest that up to 4% of the population overuse analgesics and other drugs for the treatment of pain conditions like migraine and that more than 1% of the general population in Europe, North America, and Asia suffer from medication-overuse headache (Diener & Limmroth, 2004). Treating too early can increase the risk of medication overuse in patients who often have more than one type of headache and are not able to differentiate migraine from other headache types.

Do Not Treat during the Aura Phase

A popular advice from physicians to patients with migraine attacks preceded by auras is to administer the medication during the aura phase rather than to wait until the headache has started. Although intuitively this seems wise advice, as this might prevent the subsequent headache instead of requiring to treat it, there is now good clinical evidence that this, paradoxically, will result in a reduced efficacy of triptans against the headache (Olesen *et al.*, 2004; Bates *et al.*, 1994). In these two studies triptans were found safe used during the aura, but showed reduced efficacy in treating the subsequent headache when given during the aura before the headache had started as compared to when given when the headache had already started. Thus, the clinical implication is to take a triptan only after the aura when the headache has started.

Summary

In deciding whether or not to recommend early treatment of migraine to patients, we must focus critically on the available evidence. Although early treatment intuitively would seem to be a good approach, and there are some promising results in support of early treatment, the evidence base is insufficient as yet. Some of the evidence comes from trials with inadequate designs and insufficient outcome measures, and there is a danger that the unrealistically high success rates being reported will ultimately reduce patient satisfaction because they raise expectations too high. Placebo-controlled, randomised studies within the same attack type, using sustained pain-free as the outcome measure, are required. From the clinical practice point of view we must also be aware of the potential risk of inducing medication-overuse headaches by advising all patients to treat their headaches at the very first signs of pain. On the basis of the currently available evidence, our advice to patients ought to be that they should treat their headache as soon as they are *certain* that they are developing a migraine headache, but that they should not treat during the aura phase.

References

Bates, D., *et al.* (1994). Subcutaneous sumatriptan during the migraine aura. Sumatriptan Aura Study Group. *Neurology*, 44, 1587–1592.

Burstein, R., & Jakubowski, M. (2004). Analgesic triptan action in an animal model of intracranial pain: a race against the development of central sensitization. *Annals of Neurology*, 55, 27–36.

Burstein, R., Cutrer, M.F., & Yarnitsky, D. (2000). The development of cutaneous allodynia during a migraine attack clinical evidence for the sequential recruitment of spinal and supraspinal nociceptive neurons in migraine. *Brain*, 123, 1703–1709.

Burstein, R., Collins, B., & Jakubowski, M. (2004). Defeating migraine pain with triptans: a race against the development of cutaneous allodynia. *Annals of Neurology*, 55, 19–26.

Cady, R., *et al.* (2004). Randomized, placebo-controlled comparison of early use of frovatriptan in a migraine attack versus dosing after the headache has become moderate or severe. *Current Medical Research and Opinion*, 20, 1465–1472.

Cady, R.K., *et al.* (2000). Effect of early intervention with sumatriptan on migraine pain: retrospective analyses of data from three clinical trials. *Clinical Therapeutics*, 22, 1035–1048.

Diamond, S., & Freitag, F.G. (2004). Sumatriptan 6 mg subcutaneous as a successful treatment for migraine associated with allodynia. *Neurology*, 62, A149.

Diener, H.C., & Limmroth, V. (2004). Medication-overuse headache: a worldwide problem. *Lancet Neurology*, 3, 475–483.

Dowson, A.J., *et al.* (2004). Almotriptan improves response rates when treatment is within 1 hour of migraine onset. *Headache*, 44, 318–322.

Ferrari, M.D. (2004). Should we advise patients to treat migraine attacks early? *Cephalalgia*, 24, 915–917.

Ferrari, M.D. (2005). Should we advise patients to treat migraine attacks early: methodologic issues. *European Neurology*, 53 (Suppl. 1), 17–21.

Ferrari, M.D., *et al.* (2001). Oral triptans (serotonin 5-HT(1B/1D) agonists) in acute migraine treatment: a meta-analysis of 53 trials. *Lancet*, 358, 1668–1675.

Foley, K.A., *et al.* (2005). Treating early versus treating mild: timing of migraine prescription medications among patients with diagnosed migraine. *Headache*, 45, 538–545.

Goadsby, P.J., Lipton, R.B., & Ferrari, M.D. (2002). Migraine-current understanding and treatment. *New England Journal of Medicine*, 346, 257–270.

Klapper, J., *et al.* (2004). Benefits of treating highly disabled migraine patients with zolmitriptan while pain is mild. *Cephalalgia*, 24, 918–924.

Mathew, N.T. (2003). Early intervention with almotriptan improves sustained pain-free response in acute migraine. *Headache*, 43, 1075–1079.

Mathew, N.T., Kailasam, J., & Meadors, L. (2004). Early treatment of migraine with rizatriptan: a placebo-controlled study. *Headache*, 44, 669–673.

Olesen, J., *et al.* (2004). No effect of eletriptan administration during the aura phase of migraine. *European Journal of Neurology*, 11, 671–677.

Pascual, J., & Cabarrocas, X. (2002). Within-patient early versus delayed treatment of migraine attacks with almotriptan: the sooner the better. *Headache*, 42, 28–31.

Plosker, G.L., & McTavish, D. (1994). Sumatriptan. A reappraisal of its pharmacology and therapeutic efficacy in the acute treatment of migraine and cluster headache. *Drugs*, 47, 622–651.

Scholpp, J., *et al.* (2004). Early treatment of a migraine attack while pain is still mild increases the efficacy of sumatriptan. *Cephalalgia*, 24, 925–933.

The Subcutaneous Sumatriptan International Study Group. (1991). Treatment of migraine attacks with sumatriptan. *New England Journal of Medicine*, 325, 316–321.

Tfelt-Hansen, P., *et al.* (2000). Guidelines for controlled trials of drugs in migraine: second edition. *Cephalalgia*, 20, 765–786.

Progress in Neurotherapeutics and Neuropsychopharmacology, 1:1, 63–77 © 2006 Cambridge University Press
DOI: 10.1017/S1748232105000078   Printed in the United Kingdom

Early Phase Trials of Minocycline in Amyotrophic Lateral Sclerosis

Paul H. Gordon and Joseph Choi

Department of Neurology, Columbia University, NY, USA; Email: phg8@columbia.edu

Dan H. Moore

Department of Biostatistics, California Pacific Medical Center, CA, USA; Email: dmoore@cc.UCSF.edu

Robert G. Miller

Department of Neurology, California Pacific Medical Center, CA, USA; Email: millerrx@sutterhealth.org

Key words: amyotrophic lateral sclerosis; minocycline; clinical trial; neurodegeneration.

Introduction and Overview

Amyotrophic lateral sclerosis (ALS), a neurodegenerative disease characterized by selective motor neuron cell death, leads to progressive weakness and death in an average of 3 years (Rowland & Shneider, 2001). There is no cure or known treatment that improves function. The mechanisms of motor neuron degeneration are not fully understood, but there is evidence that mitochondrial dysfunction, free radical toxicity, glutamate excitotoxicity, and intermediate filament-aggregation lead to activation of genes and enzymes that control cell death pathways, including apoptosis (Martin, 1999; Wiedemann *et al.*, 1998; Rothstein *et al.*, 1992; Hirano, 1991). Up-regulation of stress enzymes such as p38 mitogen activated protein (MAP) kinase and release of mitochondrial cytochrome *c* may contribute to activation of pro-inflammatory and pro-apoptotic modulators (Zhu *et al.*, 2002; Mota *et al.*, 2001; Horstmann *et al.*, 1998; Migheli *et al.*, 1997; Schiffer *et al.*, 1996). Inflammatory cells and cytokines, including inducible nitric oxide synthase (iNOS), components of the complement cascade, and pro-apoptotic caspase enzymes are activated in areas of neurodegeneration in ALS (Almer *et al.*, 2001; Li *et al.*, 2000; Martin *et al.*, 2000; Kostic *et al.*, 1997). Caspase enzyme inhibitors and anti-inflammatory agents slow progression in the transgenic mouse model of

Correspondence should be addressed to: Paul H. Gordon, MD, Eleanor and Lou Gehrig MDA/ALS Research Center, Neurological Institute, 710 West 168th Street, New York, NY 10032, USA; Ph: +212 305 1319; Email: phg8@columbia.edu.

ALS (Drachman *et al.*, 2002; Barneoud and Curet, 2000; Friedlander *et al.*, 1997).

Minocycline, which has both anti-inflammatory and anti-apoptotic properties, crosses the blood–brain barrier, and has been shown to have neuroprotective effects in models of ALS and other neurodegenerative disorders. This article describes the scientific evidence underlying the neuroprotective effects of minocycline, and summarizes the results of two early phase human trials of minocycline in ALS.

Purpose of the Trials

The purpose of the trials was to determine whether patients with ALS can safely tolerate moderate and high doses of minocycline over extended periods. The primary aims were to determine the safety and tolerability of minocycline in patients with ALS, including those taking riluzole, and to show whether patients with ALS can tolerate doses of up to 400 mg. The latter aim was undertaken because of the evidence of a dose–response effect in the murine model; those animals given higher doses had greater improvement in survival. Previously, doses above 200 mg/day had not been taken chronically. These trials were performed as safety, feasibility, and dose selection studies in preparation for a National Institute of Health (NIH) funded Phase III trial of efficacy, now underway.

Agent: Minocycline

Minocycline, which is approved by the Food and Drug Administration (FDA) for treatment of infection, has good central nervous system (CNS) penetration when taken orally and may inhibit cell death pathways by reducing both pro-apoptotic and pro-inflammatory enzyme activation. It has neuroprotective effects in animal models of stroke (Yrjanheikki *et al.*, 1999), trauma (Arnold *et al.*, 2001), and neurodegenerative disorders including Huntington's disease (HD) (Chen *et al.*, 2000) and Parkinson's disease (Du *et al.*, 2001).

Minocycline reduces glutamate-induced activation of microglia and interleukin production in *in vitro* models of ALS. Minocycline has been shown to reduce glutamate excitoxicity by regulating p38 pathways in cerebellar granule neuronal culture (Pi *et al.*, 2004), and prevents neurotoxicity induced by cerebrospinal fluid (CSF) from patients with motor neuron disease (Tikka *et al.*, 2002).

Several laboratories have shown that minocycline delays disease progression in the ALS transgenic mouse model (Kriz *et al.*, 2002; Van Den Bosch *et al.*, 2002; Zhu *et al.*, 2002), possibly involving down-regulation of p38 MAP Kinase. Intraperitoneal injections of 5 mg/kg/day provided an increase in lifespan of approximately 11% compared to placebo-treated mice in a blinded study of 20 superoxide dismntase-1 (SOD1) rodents (Serge Przedborski, personal communication).

In an independent laboratory, minocycline prolonged life in the ALS model (Zhu *et al.*, 2002). Mice injected with 10 mg/kg/day beginning at 5 weeks of age had delayed onset of impaired motor performance and had significantly extended survival of 11 days (9%) compared to saline-treated control mice. Pathologically, minocycline reduced the activation of caspase-1, caspase-3, iNOS and p38 MAP kinase activity secondary to upstream effects on mitochondria. It directly inhibited mitochondrial permeability-transition-mediated cytochrome *c* release, a critical early step in the activation of cell death pathways including caspase-enzyme-mediated apoptosis. The authors detected these effects *in vivo* using ALS mice and cerebral ischemia models, in neuronal cells and in isolated mitochondria.

In a separate study in the ALS mouse model, minocycline improved survival and reduced microglial activation (Van Den Bosch *et al.*, 2002). In this study, transgenic mice with the G93A human SOD1 mutation were treated every week-day with an intraperitoneal injection of saline or minocycline starting at 70 days of age. Two different minocycline doses were used: 25 and 50 mg/kg. Minocycline dose-dependently delayed decline in rotarod performance, which met statistical significance between high-dose minocycline and saline-treated mice. Mino-cycline also delayed the onset and slowed decline in muscle weakness in a dose-dependent manner, again meeting statistical significance at the 50 mg/kg dose. Both minocycline concentrations delayed mortality to significant degrees. Mice treated with the higher dose had a prolonged life span of 16%. Pathologically, at 120 days of age, mice treated with minocycline had reduced motor neuron loss, vacuolization, and microglial activation compared to control animals.

A separate laboratory also reported results of minocycline in the ALS mouse model (Kriz *et al.*, 2002). In this study, minocycline administered in the diet delayed the onset of muscle strength decline and improved survival compared to mice fed a regular diet. Pathologically, minocycline treated mice had a reduction in activation of microglia and motor neuron degeneration.

Minocycline also possesses neuroprotective properties in models of other disorders with mechanisms of cell death similar to ALS. In a rodent model of focal cerebral ischemia, minocycline reduced cortical infarction volume by 63% when started 4 h after the onset of ischemia (Yrjanheikki *et al.*, 1999). In this study, ischemia was induced by inserting nylon thread into the internal carotid artery up to the middle cerebral artery. Animals received intraperitoneal injections of minocycline at 45 mg/kg twice the first day and 22.5 mg/kg on the subsequent 2 days. Pathologic studies indicated that minocycline inhibited activation of microglia and induction of interleukin-1beta converting enzyme, and reduced cyclooxygenase-2 expression and prostaglandin E2 production.

In a study of experimental spinal cord injury in rodents, systemic administration of minocycline improved functional recovery (Arnold *et al.*, 2001). The authors reported that 90 mg/kg intraperitoneal injections 1 h following moderate spinal cord contusion provided significant improvement in motor function when compared to control animals. Those animals that received minocycline had reduced neurodegeneration, apoptosis, and caspase enzyme activation in the spinal cord.

Minocycline also prevented nigrostriatal dopaminergic neurodegeneration in the 1-methyl-4-phenyl-1,2,3,6-tetrahydropyridine (MPTP) mouse model of Parkinson's disease (Du *et al.*, 2001). In this controlled study, mice received doses of minocycline ranging from 60 to 120 mg/kg/day by oral gavage before, during and after MPTP administration. Minocycline inhibited phosphorylation of p38 MAP kinase, blocked MPTP-induced neurodegeneration and dopamine depletion, and was associated with marked reductions in iNOS and caspase-1 expression.

In a blinded study using the R6/2 HD mouse model, survival was prolonged following intraperitoneal injections of minocycline at 5 mg/kg/day (Chen *et al.*, 2000). Daily minocycline treatment beginning at 6 weeks of age significantly delayed the characteristic decline of rotarod performance and extended survival by 14% when compared to saline-treated mice. In this model there was reduction of caspase-1, and caspase-3 upregulation and of iNOS activity. There was no effect of tetracycline, which does not cross the blood–brain barrier, on performance or survival.

Comparison with Other Tetracyclines

The tetracyclines, among the first of the antibiotics to become available 50 years ago, remain widely used. Minocycline is a second-generation, long-acting tetracycline (Smilack, 1999). It is indicated in the treatment of a variety of bacterial infections, and has been used to treat brain and meningeal infections. It is a widely prescribed systemic antibiotic for the management of acne (Johnson & Nunley, 2000) and has demonstrated benefit in inflammatory arthritis (Langevitz *et al.*, 2000). Minocycline is ten times more lipid-soluble than other tetracyclines and consequently has good CNS penetration and bioavailability. The serum half-life is approximately 17 h.

Minocycline, at oral doses of 100 mg twice daily, which roughly equates to the 5 mg/kg/day doses in the SOD1 and HD models provides proven anti-inflammatory benefit in human rheumatoid arthritis. In a 2-year, double-blind protocol, minocyline was superior to hydroxychloroquine in patients with early seropositive rheumatoid arthritis (O'Dell *et al.*, 1997). Patients were significantly more likely to achieve 50% improvement and to be tapered off prednisone than controls. In blinded studies of subjects with advanced rheumatoid arthritis, 100 mg twice daily also provided statistically significant benefit when compared to control subjects (Stone *et al.*, 2003; Langevitz *et al.*, 2000).

Toxicities of minocycline are similar to those reported with other tetracyclines and include staining of dental enamel, hyperpigmentation of skin and other tissues, photosensitivity, gastrointestinal intolerance, diarrhea and vestibular side effects, including dizziness, ataxia and vertigo (Patel *et al.*, 1998). It has been reported to rarely induce immune reactions resulting in hepatitis, arthritis and drug-induced lupus, generalized hypersensitivity, serum sickness-like reactions, vasculitis, pseudotumor cerebri, hypersensitivity pneumonitis, interstitial nephritis and black thyroid syndrome (Eichenfield, 1999). The half-life is prolonged in patients with renal failure. Food and divalent cations can interfere with oral absorption. Minocycline is eliminated through the hepatobiliary and gastro-intestinal tracts. Minocycline may reduce oral contraceptive efficacy. Potentiation of warfarin-induced anticoagulation, and elevation of lithium, digoxin and theophylline levels necessitates close monitoring. The usual dosage of 100 mg every 12 h has been well tolerated in chronic use (Goulden *et al.*, 1996). In long-term therapy, periodic laboratory evaluations of organ systems, including hematopoietic, renal and hepatic studies are performed. It is contraindicated in persons who have shown hypersensitivity to any of the tetracyclines, and during pregnancy and childhood because of dental staining and interference with bone growth.

Clinical Trial

Two separate trials were conducted (Gordon *et al.*, 2004): Trial 1, at the General Clinical Research Center (GCRC) and the MDA/ALS Research Center of the University of New Mexico (UNM), and Trial 2, at the Forbes Norris MDA/ALS Research Center, California Pacific Medical Center (CPMC).

Subjects

Eligibility criteria were the same for both trials. Eligible patients were between 21 and 80 years of age, and had a diagnosis of probable or definite ALS according to modified El Escorial criteria (Brooks *et al.*, 2000). If taking riluzole, patients were on a stable dose for at least 30 days prior to enrollment. Exclusion criteria were tracheotomy ventilation; diagnosis of another concurrent neurodegenerative disease; history of renal or liver disease; history of systemic lupus erythematosis; pregnancy, lactation or being of childbearing potential and not using adequate birth control; and allergy to tetracycline antibiotics. All subjects signed informed consent approved by the individual institutional review boards.

Trial Methods

In *Trial 1*, a prospective randomized, double-blind, placebo-controlled trial, minocycline 100 mg capsules (Group 1) or identical appearing placebo (Group 2) was administered twice daily for 6 months. In *Trial 2*, a prospective, double-blind, randomized, placebo-controlled, crossover trial, minocycline (or identical appearing placebo) was administered in 50 mg tablets starting at 100 mg bid and increasing every week by 50 mg bid until reaching the highest tolerated dose or 400 mg/day. In this 8-month trial, subjects were randomized in a 3 : 1 ratio so that three of every four patients received minocycline during the first 4 months (Group 1) and then "crossed over" to placebo for the remaining 4 months. One of every four patients received placebo during the first 4 months (Group 2) and then "crossed over" to minocycline during the final 4 months. The treatment periods were chosen as sufficient to demonstrate the safety and tolerability of treatment in ALS, and to ensure that the majority of subjects completed the study.

The sample sizes consisted of 19 subjects (Trial 1) and 23 subjects (Trial 2) divided into two groups. Our primary purpose was to determine safety and tolerability of the drug during a reasonably short time period. Nineteen patients were enrolled and followed at UNM (Trial 1), 10 received drug and 9 received placebo, which provided 80% power to detect a 61% difference in the rates of adverse events (AEs) (e.g. 66% in those taking drug versus 5% in those on placebo). The cross-over design for the 23 patients enrolled and followed at CPMC (Trial 2) provided 80% power to detect a 38% difference in AEs (e.g. 33% on drug versus 5% off drug).

After providing written informed consent, and completing the baseline visit, each patient was randomly assigned to one of two treatment groups, minocycline (Group 1) or placebo (Group 2). The assignments were made by selecting the next entry from a randomization list consisting of minocycline and placebo entries placed in a random order (1 : 1 ratio Trial 1; 3 : 1 ratio Trial 2) by the GCRC biostatistician (Trial 1) and the CPMC biostatistician (DM, Trial 2) using a random number generator. The randomization assignment and drug labeling was performed by the research pharmacist at each site so that the allocation of patients was known only to them. The research pharmacist then dispensed the drugs in order to maintain blinding of the clinical teams. Following eligibility, as determined by the clinical investigator and coordinator, the patients were issued a subject identification (ID) number. This ID number was used to identify the drug for the given subject. It was also used to identify the subject's case report forms, laboratory tests, communications, and drug packages.

Outcome Measures

The primary outcome measures were the safety and tolerability measures. Information on adverse effects of medication and on intercurrent events was determined at each visit by direct questioning of the patients, clinical examination, and laboratory tests. The frequency and severity of reported AEs was recorded. Tolerability was determined by the ability to complete the study on the assigned experimental medication. Death from any cause, tracheostomy, or chronic assisted ventilation was considered a survival endpoint.

Analysis

Safety and tolerability

The total number of AEs was compared between groups using Fisher's exact test. The treatment group was compared to the control group with respect to occurrence of each type of AE. Abnormal laboratory tests were compared between the two groups using Fisher's exact test. Compliance data from medication logs and returned drug supplies was determined for each visit and by group. The number of subjects who completed the study in both groups, excluding deaths was determined in each group and compared using Fishers' exact test.

Results

Trial 1

The detailed results are given in the article by Gordon et al. (2004). Nineteen patients were enrolled in Trial 1 and randomly assigned to either Group 1 or Group 2. All were included in the intent-to-treat analysis (9 of 9 placebo, 10 of 10 minocycline). No patient was withdrawn for noncompliance, and none abandoned the trial to participate in another trial. Thirteen patients completed the full treatment course and the termination visit (6 placebo, 7 minocycline). Three patients died and three patients withdrew from the study.

Subjects were recruited for Trial 1 at the University of New Mexico between May 2001 and May 2002; the final patient completed the study in November 2002. The baseline characteristics of the patients were such that they were well matched for age, sex, weight, initial forced vital capacity (FVC), strength measures, and ALS Functional Rating Scale-Revised (ALSFRS-R) scores. There were no statistically significant differences in minor (Figure 1) or severe AEs (Figure 2) or laboratory abnormalities (Figure 3), or in the ability to complete the trial between groups. Three (2 minocycline, 1 placebo) patients died of progressive respiratory failure due to ALS. Three patients prematurely withdrew from the protocol (2 placebo, 1 minocycline) as a result of advancing weakness and inability to come to the study center. Other AEs while taking minocycline were phlebitis (1), diarrhea (1), vaginitis (1), and dyspepsia (1). No patient was withdrawn due to AEs other than death. Three patients (1 minocycline, 2 placebo) had AST/ALT elevations of less than 2.5 × normal; all were taking riluzole, which commonly elevates AST/ALT. Eight patients (3 in minocycline group, 5 in placebo group) developed mild anemia.

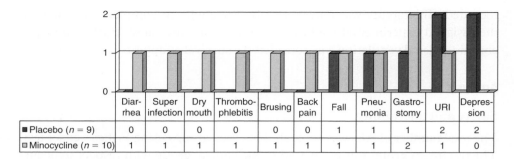

Fig. 1.
Subjects with non-serious AEs (URI, upper respiratory infection).

	Diar-rhea	Super infection	Dry mouth	Thrombo-phlebitis	Brusing	Back pain	Fall	Pneu-monia	Gastro-stomy	URI	Depres-sion
■ Placebo (*n* = 9)	0	0	0	0	0	0	1	1	1	2	2
▣ Minocycline (*n* = 10)	1	1	1	1	1	1	1	1	2	1	0

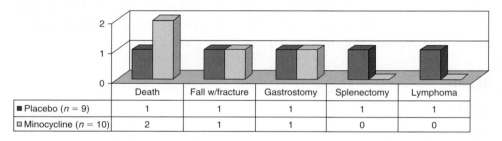

	Death	Fall w/fracture	Gastrostomy	Splenectomy	Lymphoma
■ Placebo (*n* = 9)	1	1	1	1	1
▣ Minocycline (*n* = 10)	2	1	1	0	0

Fig. 2.
Subjects with serious AEs.

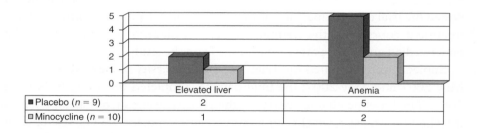

	Elevated liver	Anemia
■ Placebo (*n* = 9)	2	5
▣ Minocycline (*n* = 10)	1	2

Fig. 3.
Subjects with laboratory abnormality.

Trial 2

Twenty-three patients were enrolled in Trial 2 and randomly assigned to either Group 1 or 2. All were included in the intent-to-treat analysis. No patient was withdrawn for noncompliance, and none abandoned the trial to participate in another trial. Twenty patients completed the full course (15 in Group 1 and 5 in group 2).

Subjects were recruited at the Forbes Norris ALS Research Center, California Pacific Medical Center between June 2001 and April 2002. The final patient

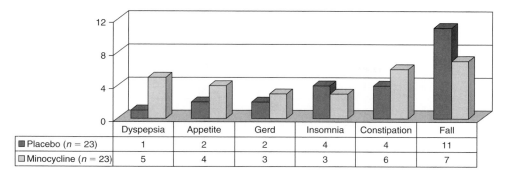

	Dyspepsia	Appetite	Gerd	Insomnia	Constipation	Fall
■ Placebo (*n* = 23)	1	2	2	4	4	11
□ Minocycline (*n* = 23)	5	4	3	3	6	7

Fig. 4.
Adverse events.

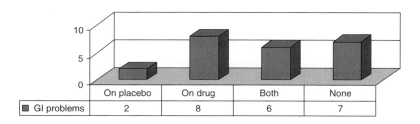

	On placebo	On drug	Both	None
■ GI problems	2	8	6	7

Fig. 5.
Gastrointestinal AEs (*p* = 0.057).

completed the trial in January 2003. The baseline characteristics of the patients were well matched for age, sex, weight, initial FVC, and ALSFRS-R scores.

Analysis of the primary outcome, the safety and tolerability data, showed that there was a trend toward increased gastrointestinal symptoms overall while taking the higher doses of minocycline compared to placebo ($p = 0.057$) (Figures 4 and 5). Individual AEs were not significantly different. Common AEs while taking minocycline were constipation (6), dyspepsia (5), appetite loss (4), and reflux (3). Three patients dropped out (1 while taking minocycline, 2 while taking placebo) due to gastrostomy placement (1), move out of state (1), and personal reasons (1). There was no significant difference in the dropout rate while taking drug compared to placebo, and there were no deaths. Elevations of BUN ($p < 0.05$) and ALT/AST ($p < 0.05$) while taking minocycline were statistically significant, but were not considered to be clinically significant. Figure 6 shows the changes that occurred in laboratory values while taking drug and while taking placebo. Twenty-one of twenty-three patients took riluzole throughout the trial. However, riluzole alone could not account for the changes in laboratory data due to the cross-over design. Other laboratory measures were unchanged in each group. Nineteen of twenty-three patients tolerated the target dose of minocycline; the maximum mean tolerated dose was 387 mg/day.

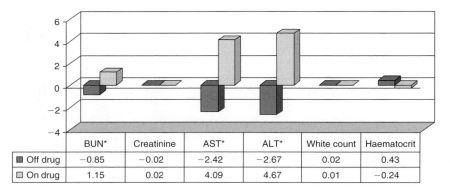

	BUN*	Creatinine	AST*	ALT*	White count	Haematocrit
■ Off drug	−0.85	−0.02	−2.42	−2.67	0.02	0.43
☐ On drug	1.15	0.02	4.09	4.67	0.01	−0.24

Fig. 6.
Change in laboratory results (*$p = 0.01$*).

Conclusions

These were the first controlled trials of minocycline, which probably acts by reducing the activation of enzymes involved in cell death pathways, in human ALS. There is laboratory evidence that minocycline inhibits cytochrome *c* release, reduces the activation of p38 MAP kinase, and down-regulates pro-apoptotic caspase enzymes and pro-inflammatory mediators. It slows progression in animal models of neurodegenerative disorders, and has high CNS penetration when taken orally (Smilack, 1999). Minocycline has been shown to be effective in long-term use for the treatment of inflammatory arthritis (Langevitz *et al.*, 2000), and has been administered safely for extended periods for the treatment of acne (Goulden *et al.*, 1996). The purpose of the trials was to test the safety and tolerability of minocycline over prolonged periods in subjects with ALS taking riluzole (Trial 1) and to test doses of minocycline higher than previously given, attempting to obtain the highest possible CNS levels (Trial 2). The latter was undertaken because of the appearance of a dose–response effect in SOD1 model studies in which higher doses provided greater neuroprotective benefit (Van Den Bosch *et al.*, 2002). These trials were designed as safety, feasibility, and dose-selection studies in planning for a larger Phase III trial of efficacy.

Subjects tolerated the combination of riluzole and minocycline over 6 months in Trial 1. The occurrence of AEs was similar between placebo and intervention groups. The majority of patients could tolerate higher than standard doses in Trial 2, although gastrointestinal side effects became more prominent, and liver and renal function measures were elevated at the higher doses (Gordon *et al.*, 2004). Allowing patients to take the highest tolerated dose instead of fixed doses may have minimized dropout rates because several patients were not able to take 400 mg/day. Consequently, the Phase III trial was similarly designed to allow patients to take their maximally tolerated dose.

Influence on the Field

Since publication of the early phase human trials, research into the potential neuroprotective effects of minocycline has continued to appear in the literature, both from clinical and basic research studies. Minocycline is now being tested in a series of NIH-driven Phase II futility trials assessing different agents in Parkinson's disease and has been tested in early phase human trials in HD.

Not all of the laboratory studies have been positive, however. In one study, seven MPTP-exposed cynomolgus monkeys were given either IV (0.2 mg/kg) or oral (200 mg bid) minocycline (Diguet *et al.*, 2004). Minocycline treated animals tended to have more severe parkinsonism and had greater loss of putaminal dopaminergic nerve endings. The same laboratory also showed worsening in a HD model. However, most published reports continue to be positive. Recent experiments have shown that minocycline acts as a neuroprotective agent in models of HIV/AIDS (Zink *et al.*, 2005), Down's syndrome (Hunter *et al.*, 2004), Alzheimer's disease (Ryu *et al.*, 2004), and multiple sclerosis (Popovic *et al.*, 2002).

The scientific study of minocycline now includes trials in combination with other agents. In ALS models, several laboratories have now shown that minocycline may have additive neuroprotective effects when given with other drugs. Minocycline in combination with riluzole and nimodipine was shown to extent survival in the murine model (Kriz *et al.*, 2003), and one laboratory showed that a combination of minocycline and creatine resulted in additive benefit in the model (Zhang *et al.*, 2003). In this study, mice were fed a diet supplemented with 2% creatine, and were injected with 22 mg/kg/day of minocycline intraperitoneally. Monotherapy and untreated control groups were fed control diet or injected with saline. Minocycline alone extended survival approximately 13%; creatine 12%; and the combination 25% (Zhang *et al.*, 2003). Similarly, minocycline in combination with either glatiramer acetate (Guiliani *et al.*, 2005b) or beta interferon (Guiliani *et al.*, 2005a) provided additive effects in a model of multiple sclerosis.

Translation to Clinical Practice

Despite advances in understanding of the pathogenesis, ALS remains an essentially untreatable disease. Riluzole is the only currently approved treatment for ALS, but its effect prolongs life only 2 months on average (Lacomblez *et al.*, 1996). Given the myriad mechanisms of neurodegeneration, it is likely that agents that target different processes such as minocycline may have a more meaningful effect, and minocycline may eventually prove to be a good candidate for testing in human trials of combinations of agents.

The small sample size and limited duration of the trials described here renders it premature to draw conclusions regarding efficacy and, because of the abnormalities detected in liver and renal function while taking minocycline in combination with riluzole, along with the conflicting basic science data, we do not consider it appropriate to recommend prescription of minocycline for treatment of ALS. The tolerability of minocycline in these trials was acceptable, which, along with the body of positive basic science data, supports proceeding to a larger Phase III trial in ALS. The Phase III trial began in November 2003 and is testing the highest tolerated dose of minocycline up to 400 mg/day. The trial is 80% powered ($\alpha = 0.05$) to detect an 18% change in the rate of deterioration of the ALSFRS-R over 13 months. A total of 400 patients will be enrolled at 30 centers across the US (http://clinicaltrials.gov/ct/show/NCT00047723?order=1). The ALSFRS-R was chosen as the primary outcome because it measures function, something patients may find more meaningful than survival, and because it can be administered over the telephone, thereby reducing dropout compared to outcomes that require patients to attend the clinic.

Treatment of ALS

Practice Parameters, published by the American Academy of Neurology, provide guidance in the care of patients with ALS (Miller *et al.*, 1999). Approximately 60% of ALS patients in the USA take riluzole. The remaining do not because the drug is very expensive and not covered by their health plan, because of side effects, or because they or their doctors are unimpressed by the modest prolongation in survival it offers (Bradley *et al.*, 2004). Other important aspects of ALS care are the palliative treatments offered by multi-disciplinary ALS clinics, where patients can be evaluated and treated by multiple therapists and specialists trained in caring for the disorder in a single morning or afternoon. The expertise offered in these clinics helps patients maintain function and independence to the extent possible. Gastrostomy for those with dysphagia and non-invasive ventilation for those with respiratory insufficiency help relieve symptoms, improve quality of life and may prolong survival (Miller *et al.*, 1999). Approximately 5% of patients eventually choose to have tracheostomy and mechanical ventilation, which can extend survival indefinitely despite continuing disease progression. The close monitoring offered in the clinics is accentuated in patients who participate in clinical research, which generally requires patients to visit the center every month or every other month. While palliative care can help improve quality of life for ALS patients, better treatments will come through the design of robust clinical trials testing agents with strong scientific justification such as minocycline.

Acknowledgement

Supported by GCRC grant number M01 RR00997.

References

Almer, G., Guegan, C., Teismann, P., Naini, A., et al. (2001). Increased expression of the proinflammatory enzyme cyclooxygenase-2 in amyotrophic lateral sclerosis. *Annals of Neurology*, 49, 176–185.

Arnold, P.M., Ameenuddin, S., Citron, B.A., SantaCruz, K.S., Qin, F., & Festoff, B.W. (2001). *Systemic Administration of Minocycline Improves Functional Recovery and Morphometric Analysis After Spinal Cord Injury (SCI)*. San Diego, CA: Society for Neuroscience, November 2001 [Abstract 769.4].

Barneoud, P., & Curet, O. (2000). Beneficial effects of lysine acetylsalicylate, a soluble salt of aspirin, on motor performance in a transgenic model of amyotrophic lateral sclerosis. *Experimental Neurology*, 155, 243–251.

Bradley, W.G., Anderson, F., Gowda, N., Miller, R.G., & ALS CARE Study Group. (2004). Changes in the management of ALS since the publication of the AAN ALS practice parameter 1999. *Amyotrophic Lateral Sclerosis and Other Motor Neuronal Disorders*, 5, 240–244.

Brooks, B.R., Miller, R.G., Swash, M., Munsat, T.L., for the world federation of neurology research group on motor neuron diseases. (2000). El Escorial revisited: revised criteria for the diagnosis of amyotrophic lateral sclerosis. *Amyotrophic Lateral Sclerosis and Other Motor Neuronal Disorders*, 557–560.

Chen, M., Ona, V.O., Li, M., Ferrante, R.J., Fink, K.B., Zhu, S., Bian, J., et al. (2000). Minocycline inhibits caspase-1 and caspase-3 expression and delays mortality in a transgenic mouse model of Huntington disease. *Nature Medicine*, 6, 797–801.

Diguet, E., Fernagut, P.O., Wei, X., Du, Y., et al. (2004). Deleterious effects of minocycline in animal models of Parkinson disease and Huntington disease. *European Journal of Neuroscience*, 19, 3266–3276.

Drachman, D.B., Frank, K., Dykes-Hoberg, M., Teismann, P., Almer, G., Przedborski, S., & Rothstein, J.D. (2002). Cyclooxygenase 2 inhibition protects motor neurons and prolongs survival in a transgenic mouse model of ALS. *Annals of Neurology*, 52, 771–778.

Du, Y., Ma, Z., Lin, S., Dodel, R.C., Goa, F., Bales, K.R., et al. (2001). Minocycline prevents nigrostriatal dopaminergic neurodegeneration in the MPTP model of Parkinson's disease. *Proceedings of the National Academy of Science*, 98, 14669–14674.

Eichenfield, A.H. (1999). Minocycline and autoimmunity. *Current Opinion in Pediatrics*, 11, 447–456.

Friedlander, R.M., Brown, R.H., Gagliardini, V., Wang, J., & Yuan, J. (1997). Inhibition of ICE slows amyotrophic lateral sclerosis in mice. *Nature*, 388, 31.

Gordon, P.H., Moore, D.H., Gelinas, D.F., Qualls, C., Meister, M.E., Werner, J., Mendoza, M., Mass, J., Kushner, G., & Miller, R.G. (2004). Placebo Controlled Phase I/II studies of minocycline in amyotrophic lateral sclerosis. *Neurology*, 62, 1845–1847.

Goulden, V., Glass, D., & Cunliffe, W.J. (1996). Safety of long-term high-dose minocycline in the treatment of acne. *British Journal of Dermatology*, 134, 693–695.

Guiliani, F., Fu, S.A., Metz, L.M., & Yong, V.W. (2005a). Effective combination of minocycline and interferon-beta in a model of multiple sclerosis. *Journal of Neuroimmunology*, 165, 83–91.

Guiliani, F., Metz, L.M., Wilson, T., Fan, Y., Bar-Or, A., & Yong, V.W. (2005b). Additive effect of the combination of glatiramer acetate and minocycline in a model of MS. *Journal of Neuroimmunology*, 158, 213–221.

Hirano, A. (1991). Cytopathology in amyotrophic lateral sclerosis. *Advances in Neurology*, 56, 91–101.

Horstmann, S., Kahle, P.J., & Borasio, G.D. (1998). Inhibitors of p38 mitogen-activated protein kinase promote neuronal survival *in vitro*. *Journal of Neuroscience Research*, 52, 483–490.

Hunter, C.L., Bachman, D., & Granholm, A.C. (2004). Minocycline prevents cholinergic loss in a mouse model of Down's syndrome. *Annals of Neurology*, 56, 675–688.

Johnson, B.A., & Nunley, J.R. (2000). Topical therapy for acne vulgaris. *Postgraduation Medicine*, 107, 69–80.

Kostic, V., Jackson-Lewis, V., de Bilbao, F., Dubois-Dauphin, M., & Przedborski, S. (1997). Bcl-2: prolonging life in a transgenic mouse model of familial amyotrophic lateral sclerosis. *Science*, 277, 559–562.

Kriz, J., Gowing, G., & Julien, J.P. (2003). Efficient three-drug cocktail for disease induced by mutant superoxide dismutase. *Annals of Neurology*, 53, 429–436.

Kriz, J., Nguyen, M., & Julien, J. (2002). Minocycline slows disease progression in a mouse model of amyotrophic lateral sclerosis. *Neurobiological Disease*, 10, 268.

Lacomblez, L., Bensimon, G., Leigh, P.N., Guillet, P., & Meininger, V. (1996). Dose-ranging study of riluzole in amyotrophic lateral sclerosis. Amyotrophic Lateral Sclerosis/Riluzole Study Group II. *Lancet*, 347, 1425–1431.

Langevitz, P., Livneh, A., Bank, I., & Pras, M. (2000). Benefits and risks of minocycline in rheumatoid arthritis. *Drug Safety*, 22, 405–414.

Li, M., Ona, V.O., Guegan, C., Chen, M., Jackson-Lewis, V., Andrews, L.J., Olszewski, A.J., et al. (2000). Functional role of caspase-1 and caspase-3 in an ALS transgenic mouse model. *Science*, 288, 335–339.

Martin, L.J. (1999). Neuronal death in amyotrophic lateral sclerosis is apoptosis: possible contribution of a programmed cell death mechanism. *Journal of Neuropathology Experimental Neurology*, 58, 459–471.

Martin, L.J., Price, A.C., Kaiser, A., Shaikh, A.Y., & Liu, Z. (2000). Mechanisms for neuronal degeneration in amyotrophic lateral sclerosis and in models of motor neuron death. *International Journal of Molecular Medicine*, 5, 3–13.

Migheli, A., Piva, R., Atzori, C., Troost, D., & Schiffer, D. (1997). c-Jun, JNK/SAPk kinases and transcription factor NF-kB are selectively activated in astrocytes, but not motor neurons, in amyotrophic lateral sclerosis. *Journal of Neuropathology and Experimental Neurology*, 56, 1314–1322.

Miller, R.G., Rosenberg, J.A., Gelinas, D.F., Mitsumoto, H., et al. (1999). Practice parameter: the care of the patient with amyotrophic lateral sclerosis (an evidence-based review): report of the Quality Standards Subcommittee of the American Academy of Neurology: ALS Practice Parameters Task Force. *Neurology*, 52, 1311–1323.

Mota, M., Reeder, M., Chernoff, J., & Bazenet, C.E. (2001). Evidence for a role of mixed lineage kinases in neuronal apoptosis. *Journal of Neuroscience*, 21, 4949–4957.

O'Dell, J.R., Haire, C.E., Palmer, et al. (1997). Treatment of early rheumatoid arthritis with minocycline or placebo: results of a randomized, double blind, placebo-controlled trial. *Arthritis Rheumatology*, 40, 842–848.

Patel, K., Chishire, D., & Vance, A. (1998). Oral and systemic effects of prolonged minocycline therapy. *British Dental Journal*, 185, 560–562.

Pi, R., Li, W., Lee, N.T., Chan, H.H., et al. (2004). Minocycline prevents glutamate-induced apoptosis of cerebellar granule neurons by differential regulation of p38 and Akt pathways. *Journal of Neurochemistry*, 91, 1219–1230.

Popovic, N., Schubart, A., Goetz, B.D., Zhang, S.C., Linington, C., & Duncan, I.D. (2002). Inhibition of autoimmune encephalomyelitis by a tetracycline. *Annals of Neurology*, 52, 215–223.

Rothstein, J.D., Martin, L.J., & Kuncl, R.W. (1992). Decreased glutamate transport by the brain and spinal cord in amyotrophic lateral sclerosis. *New England Journal of Medicine*, 236, 1464–1468.

Rowland, L.P., & Shneider, N.A. (2001). Amyotrophic lateral sclerosis. *New England Journal of Medicine*, 344, 1688–1700.

Ryu, J.K., Franciosi, S., Sattayaprasert, P., Kim, S.U., & McLarnon, J.G. (2004). Minocycline inhibits neuronal death and glial activation induced by beta-amyloid peptide in rat hippocampus. *Glia*, 48, 85–90.

Schiffer, D., Cordera, S., Cavalla, P., & Migheli, A. (1996). Reactive astro-gliosis of the spinal cord in amyotrophic lateral sclerosis. *Journal of Neurological Science*, 139, 27–33.

Smilack, J.D. (1999). The Tetracyclines. *Mayo Clinical Proceedings*, 74, 727–729.

Stone, M., Fortin, P.R., Pacheco-Tena, C., & Inman, R.D. (2003). Should tetracycline treatment be used more extensively for rheumatoid arthritis? Metaanalysis demonstrates clinical benefit with reduction in disease activity. *Journal of Rheumatology*, 30, 2112–2122.

Tikka, T.M., Vartiainen, N.E., Goldsteins, G., Oja, S.S., Andersen, P.M., Marklund, S.L., & Koistinaho, J. (2002). Minocycline prevents neurotoxicity induced by cerebrospinal fluid from patients with motor neurone disease. *Brain*, 125, 722–731.

Van Den Bosch, L., Tillkin, P., Lemmens, G., & Robberecht, W. (2002). Minocycline delays disease onset and mortality in a transgenic model of ALS. *Neuroreport*, 13, 1067–1070.

Wiedemann, F., Winkler, K., Juznetsoc, A., *et al.* (1998). Impairment of mitochondrial function in skeletal muscle of patients with amyotrophic lateral sclerosis. *Journal of Neurological Science*, 156, 65–72.

Yrjanheikki, J., Tikka, T., Keinanen, R., Goldsteins, G., Chan, P.H., & Koistinaho, J. (1999). A tetracycline derivative, minocycline, reduces inflammation and protects against focal cerebral ischemia with a wide therapeutic window. *Proceedings of the National Academy of Science*, 96, 13496–13500.

Zhang, W., Narayanan, M., & Friedlander, R.M. (2003). Additive neuroprotective effects of minocycline with creatine in a mouse model of ALS. *Annals of Neurology*, 53, 267–270.

Zhu, S., Stravrovskaya, I.G., Drozda, M., *et al.* (2002). Minocycline inhibits cytochrome *c* release and delays progression of amyotrophic lateral sclerosis in mice. *Nature*, 417, 74–78.

Zink, M.C., Uhrlaub, J., DeWitt, J., Voelker, T., Bullock, B., *et al.* (2005). Neuroprotective and anti-human immunodeficiency virus activity of minocycline. *Journal of the American Medical Association*, 293, 2003–2011.

Progress in Neurotherapeutics and Neuropsychopharmacology, 1:1, 79–90 © 2006 Cambridge University Press
DOI: 10.1017/S174823210500008X   Printed in the United Kingdom

Creatine as a Potential Treatment for Amyotrophic Lateral Sclerosis

---

Jeremy M. Shefner

Department of Neurology, SUNY Upstate Medical University, Syracuse, New York, NY, USA;
Email: SHEFNERJ@upstate.edu

Key words: Creatine; amyotrophic lateral sclerosis; clinical trials; neurotherapeutics; transgenic mouse models; ALS functional rating scale.

Introduction

Amyotrophic lateral sclerosis (ALS) is a rare degenerative disorder of large motor neurons that results in progressive wasting and paralysis of voluntary muscles of the extremities, bulbar regions and respiratory apparatus (Rowland, 1994; Mulder, 1982). The incidence of ALS is currently approximately 2/100 000/year (Chio & Silani, 2001; Haverkamp *et al.*, 1995) with a prevalence of approximately 5/100 000. The lifetime ALS risk is 1 in 600 to 1 in 1000. Fifty percent of ALS cases die within 3 years of onset of symptoms and 90% die within 5 years (Shefner, 1996; Kurtzke & Kurland, 1989). The median age of onset is 55 years. In sporadic disease, males are at slightly greater risk, while the male/female ratio is 1 : 1 in most cases of familial disease. Ten Percent of patients have a history of the disease in first degree relatives; about 20% of these patients have a mutation in the gene encoding cytosolic copper–zinc superoxide dismutase (SOD1) have been robustly identified as causing typical familial ALS (fALS) (Rosen *et al.*, 1993).

Patients with ALS typically present with focal weakness of an arm, a leg, or of facial and bulbar muscles. The weakness typically progresses regionally and ultimately involves all muscles of voluntary movement. Both lower motor neurons (spinal) and upper (cortical) motor neurons are involved, so that patients display signs of atrophy, fasciculations, cramps and weakness in combination with spasticity, increased stretch reflexes and incoordination. Although there is sometimes pathologic evidence of sensory neuron loss, clinically, sensory signs are sparse or absent (Shefner *et al.*, 1991). There is relative sparing of muscles of eye movement

Correspondence should be addressed to: Jeremy M. Shefner, MD, PhD, Department of Neurology, SUNY Upstate Medical University, Syracuse, New york, NY, USA. Email: SHEFNERJ@upstate.edu

and the urinary sphincters. Natural history studies have determined that age at onset, site of onset, delay from first symptom to diagnosis and rate of change in respiratory function and functional rating scales are the significant covariates of survival (Teaynor *et al.*, 2004; Jablecki *et al.*, 1989; Kurtzke, 1989; Gubbay *et al.*, 1985).

The first demonstration that the disease course in ALS could be altered by pharmacologic intervention was in 1994, when riluzole was shown to prolong survival in a trial of 155 patients with ALS (Bensimon *et al.*, 1994). This finding was confirmed in a second and larger study (Lacomblez *et al.*, 1996); since then, more than a dozen clinical trials have failed to demonstrate efficacy of a variety of experimental agents (Carter *et al.*, 2003; Cudkowicz *et al.*, 2003; Andreassen *et al.*, 2000; Eisen & Weber, 1999; Gredal *et al.*, 1997; Lai *et al.*, 1997; Group A-CTS, 1996; Miller *et al.*, 1996). These agents have been directed towards glutamate homeostasis, apoptosis, oxidative stress and neuroprotection. All of these trials were based on evidence of potential efficacy in animal or *in vitro* models. In these pre-clinical models, a relationship has been established between abnormalities in glutamate transport and ALS-specific motor neuron death (Rothstein *et al.*, 2005, 1996; Trotti *et al.*, 1999; Rothstein, 1996). Oxidative stress (Robberecht, 2000; Ferrante *et al.*, 1997) also has been shown to contribute to neuronal death both in experimentals and in tissue from ALS patients. Neurofilament aggregation, production and degradation is abnormal as well (Julien *et al.*, Julien & Mushynski, 1998; Rouleau *et al.*, 1996). All of these potential disease mechanisms provide targets for disease intervention, but none as yet has provided a pathway for successful therapy.

Abnormalities in mitochondrial function have been demonstrated in ALS patients and models. Tissue from ALS patients shows mitochondrial abnormalities in both neural and non-neural tissue, including in otherwise normal appearing corticomotor neurons (Sasaki & Iwata, 1999; Hirano, 1991; Nakano *et al.*, 1987; Masui *et al.*, 1985). Mitochondrial DNA mutations have been found with increasing frequency, especially in older individuals; one such mutation is strongly associated with sporadic ALS (Ro *et al.*, 2003). In transgenic mice bearing a human point mutation in SOD1 causing fALS in mice, mitochondrial swelling and vacuolization are seen prior to symptom onset in two genetically distinct strains (Kong & Xu, 1998; Bruijn *et al.*, 1997; Dal Canto, 1995; Wong *et al.*, 1995). Prior to disease onset, abundant abnormal mitochondria were noted in motor axons from fALS mice. Disease onset correlated with massive mitochondrial vacuolation, which decreased as disease progressed. Motor axons remained viable, however, until well after the development of weakness.

A number of strategies have been considered to protect mitochondria from damage in ALS. Creatine kinase was conceived as a potential treatment because of its ability to provide an intracellular energy buffering and transport system, which connects sites of energy production (mitochondria) with sites of energy consumption (Hemmer & Walliman, 1993). Relevant neuroprotective mechanisms by which creatine might act include the regeneration of cytoplasmic ATP by phosphocreatine. This regenerated ATP is then utilized by sodium potassium ATPase to maintain membrane potential and by calcium ATPase for calcium buffering. Creatine administration also blocks the mitochondrial transition pore. The mitochondrial transition pore is an opening of the inner mitochondrial membrane, which occurs in response to a variety of stimuli including elevations in mitochondrial calcium as well as oxidative stress (Beutner *et al.*, 1998). The opening of the mitochondrial transition pore has been linked to both excitotoxic and apoptotic cell death (Schinder *et al.*, 1996; White & Reynolds, 1996).

In the fALS mouse, numerous studies have shown that creatine administration prolongs survival (Klivenyi *et al.*, 2004; Zhang *et al.*, 2003; Klivenyi *et al.*, 1999; Brown *et al.*, 1988). Given alone, creatine was either equally effective (Snow *et al.*, 2003), or significantly more effective (Klivenyi *et al.*, 1999) than riluzole in this model. Its benefit was additive with other neuroprotective agents in some studies (Klivenyi *et al.*, 2004; Zhang *et al.*, 2003) but not others (Snow *et al.*, 2003).

In summary, ample preclinical evidence supports the study of creatine in humans with ALS. Creatine was felt to be safe, based on prior experience with both athletes and patients with a variety of muscle diseases. Based on these data, we conducted a randomized, placebo-controlled trial of creatine in patients with ALS. In doing so, we addressed a number of difficulties related to the experimental use of a readily available compound in a progressive, ultimately fatal disease. A crucial question was whether patients would be willing to participate in such a trial, given their ability to obtain the substance at low cost at grocery stores, pharmacies or health food stores. We discussed this question with a sample of ALS patients at a single large ALS clinic. Perhaps surprisingly, the consensus was that, if the trial were short, many patients were willing to participate. Another question was whether patients would compliant with respect to not taking additional creatine during the study. This was assessed using measurements of urinary creatine.

Methods

This study was performed by members of the Northeast ALS Clinical Trials Consortium. Subjects were randomized in a 1 : 1 fashion to receive treatment for 6 months with creatine monohydrate (supplied by Avicena Group) at a dose of 20 g/day for 5 days followed by 5 g/day, or matching placebo. The 6-month trial period was chosen to maximize patient compliance. All study personnel were blind to treatment assignment throughout the study. An independent Safety Monitoring Committee (SMC) reviewed the safety data every 3 months throughout the study.

Eligible participants, 18 to 80 years of age, had a clinical diagnosis of definite or probable ALS (Brooks, 1994), a Functional Vital Capacity (FVC) greater than or equal to 50% predicted and disease duration of 5 years or less. As change in arm strength was the primary outcome measure, upper extremity strength had to be sufficient so that at least four of eight muscle groups could be evaluated using the quantitative isometric strength apparatus. Subjects could take riluzole if the dose was stable for at least 2 months prior to the baseline visit.

Subjects were seen monthly throughout the active treatment phase of the trial. At each visit, adverse events were noted and all measurements of all primary and secondary outcome measures occurred. This included quantitative isometric muscle strength evaluation of eight upper extremity muscles, global function as assessed by the ALS Functional Rating Scale (Cedarbaum *et al.*, 1999), and motor unit number estimation of a single hand intrinsic muscle. Safety blood and urine tests were performed at baseline, 3 and 6 months and included blood creatinine and Blood Urea Nitrogen (BUN) and urine glucose and protein. Urine for creatine measurement was collected at 3 months from a 24-hour urine collection. Deaths (or tracheostomy) were reported as they occurred: either event was considered a survival endpoint.

Prior to any site enrolling patients into this trial, formal training was provided to all sites on performance of outcome measures. For MVIC and MUNE, variability of measurement on four normal control subjects was assessed, with a criterion for acceptable intra-rater variability set at less than 15% for MVIC and 20% for MUNE.

Statistical Analysis

The sample size was based on the slope of the expected average decline in arm strength. For 102 subjects, with 51 patients per group, power analysis showed an 80% chance of detecting a 50% decrease in the rate of decline at a two sided significance level of $p = 0.05$. Preliminary values for the rate of decline and its standard deviation were obtained from prior studies (Cudkowicz *et al.*, 2003; Miller *et al.*, 2001). A total of 104 patients were recruited into the study; 19 patients did not complete the study (6 patients in active treatment, 13 in placebo), with 8 study dropouts due to death.

The statistical analyses were performed according to the intention-to-treat principle. Analysis of the primary outcome variable used a mixed model analysis of variance (Cudkowicz *et al.*, 2003). Strength measured from all muscles was combined by averaging normalized data to create a single number called a megascore. The dependent variable was the slope of the patient's arm megascore measured at baseline and months 1 through 6. The independent variables were treatment, time and a time-treatment interaction. The intercept and time variables were also modeled as random effects. The above analysis was repeated for both the ALS Functional Rating Scale and for motor unit number estimation.

Results

One hundred and four patients were enrolled from 14 centers. Fifty subjects were enrolled in the creatine group and 54 in placebo. Randomization was successful in ensuring that no statistically significant differences were present in any baseline measure between treatment and placebo groups. Fifty percent of patients in the placebo group were on riluzole, as compared to 54% for the active treatment group. Pre-treatment demographic information is presented in Table 1.

No significant change was noted between placebo and treatment groups for any of the primary or secondary outcome measures: the decline over time is shown for strength, ALS-FRS and MUNE in Figures 1–3. Of the eight deaths observed on study, six were in the placebo group and two were in the creatine group. This difference was also not significant.

Compliance as assessed by urinary creatine levels was good but not perfect. At baseline, only 1 of 68 subjects who had urine obtained at both baseline and 3 month showed a urinary creatine concentration of more than 0.5 g/l at baseline. However, 6 of the 31 subjects in the placebo group who supplied urine collections had urine creatine concentrations of greater than 0.5 g/l at the 3-month time point. Conversely, however, 6 of 37 subjects in the creatine group had urinary creatine concentrations of less than 0.5 g/l at 3 months, indicating similar amounts of non-compliance in both treatment and placebo groups.

Safety

Creatine was well tolerated. Weight declined at an equal rate for both groups and there were no abnormal values on blood testing for either group. Thirty one serious adverse events were reported; all were felt to be due to disease progression and none occurred more frequently in the treatment group as compared to the placebo group.

Table 1. **Baseline Characteristics**

	CREATINE	PLACEBO
N	50	54
Age	59(12.5)	59(10.8)
Weight (kg)	77.1(17.7)	79.2(16.3)
BMI	22.4(4)	23.2(4.3)
FVC (%)	85(17.2)	84(22.3)
Time from symptom onset (y)	1.7(1.1)	2.2(1.1)
Sex (M/F)	33/17	31/23
Onset (Limb/Bulbar)	40/10	38/16
Family History (No/Yes)	49/1	51/3
MVIC (Z)	0.86(1.1)	0.70(1.0)
ALS-FRS-R	42(5.3)	41(5.9)
MUNE	60(26.6)	57(24.9)

Values with standard deviations in parenthesis.

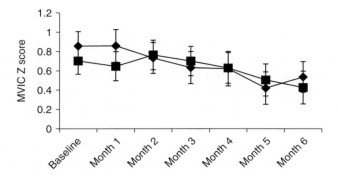

Fig. 1.

Change in MVIC Arm Z score over time in patients treated with placebo (solid squares) and with creatine (solid diamonds). Vertical bars represent standard error of the mean.

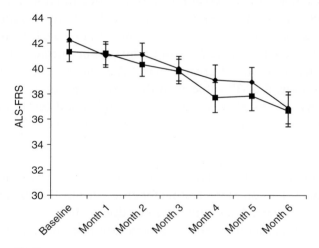

Fig. 2.

Change in ALS-FRS-R scores over time in patients treated with placebo (solid squares) and with creatine (solid diamonds). Vertical bars represent standard error of the mean.

Interpretation of Results as a Futility Analysis

This study was powered only to detect a 50% or greater change in the rate of progression of ALS. As such, the failure to show a significant positive effect of treatment might have limited clinical significance. However, the power of a study can only be estimated prior to study performance, based on data from previous investigations. Once data are acquired, confidence intervals can be applied to place an upper boundary of the size of any real effect for any given outcome measure. For the four outcome measures MVIC, Grip strength, ALS-FRS-R and MUNE, 95% confidence intervals were generated around the change in slope between placebo and treatment groups. Based on this analysis, we can conclude with 95%

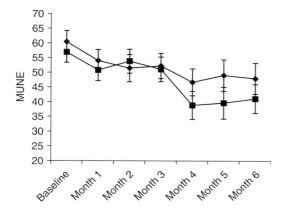

Fig. 3.
Change in MUNE over time in patients treated with placebo (solid squares) and with creatine (solid diamonds). Vertical bars represent standard error of the mean.

confidence that the true reduction in slope due to creatine treatment was less than 23% for arm strength, 19% for handgrip, 48% for ALS-FRS and 38% for MUNE. Thus, despite the lack of power estimated at the start of the study, the results obtained allow for an estimate size of a true beneficial effect of creatine that is less than the level for which the study was initially powered.

Discussion

In this study, creatine at a dose of 5 g daily was well tolerated by ALS patients, but failed to show benefit over a 6-month period. Our finding is in accord with another recently reported study (Groeneveld *et al.*, 2003), in which creatine at 10 g daily also showed no benefit. However, these results are in direct conflict with the efficacy noted in multiple animal trials using the fALS mouse model, where creatine was effective both alone and in combination with other agents. There are at least three possible reasons for this discrepancy. The most obvious possibility is that the fALS mouse model does not accurately reflect processes crucial to disease progression in human sporadic ALS. The one drug shown to have a positive effect on survival in ALS patients is riluzole, which also prolongs life in the fALS model (Schiefer *et al.*, 2002; Gurney *et al.*, 1998). However, other drugs such as celecoxib and gabapentin have been modestly to markedly effective in the mouse, but have not shown efficacy in humans (Klivenyi *et al.*, 2004; Drachman *et al.*, 2002; Gurney *et al.*, 1996).

Before making the conclusion that preclinical models of ALS are inadequate however, issues of dosing and central nervous system (CNS) penetration are important to address. With respect to directly comparing the human and mouse data, the two biggest differences in study design have to do with timing of drug administration and dosage. When fALS mice were fed a diet that was 2% creatine, life was prolonged by 26 days (Klivenyi *et al.*, 1999) with a significant effect also noted with 1% creatine. These doses are of the same order of magnitude as those used in the current study as well as the recently reported study using 10 g daily. However, since mice consume much more daily calories per unit weight than do humans, it is likely that the creatine dose used here is somewhat lower than the equivalent mouse dose shown to be effective. In addition creatine treatment in the mouse was started at day 70 of life, approximately 50 days prior to disease onset in the animals used. Such a treatment schedule in humans would require treating patients 10–20 years prior to the development of ALS-related symptoms. Early treatment of mice was also employed in studies using celecoxib and gabapentin. More recent therapeutic studies in the fALS mouse have initiated treatment at disease onset, which may provide results more directly applicable to human trials.

Another possible explanation for the lack of efficacy noted in this trial, as well as other recent ALS trials, is that human trials are significantly underpowered to detect modest therapeutic effects. Given the constraints imposed by the fact the creatine was readily available and felt by the ALS patient community to be benign, use of a sample of 100 patients studied for a relatively short period was the only practical way to perform this study. However, the inevitable result is that a small positive effect would be unlikely to be detected. Based on survival studied, the beneficial effect of riluzole is an, approximately 10% increase in total survival after diagnosis. Benefits of this magnitude may be significant if they prove additive with other agents, but studies of the size and duration reported here are unlikely to detect such effects. If the goal of future studies is to detect modest beneficial effects of therapeutic agents, larger sample sizes and longer study duration are likely to be necessary.

Finally, it should be noted that this study and most other recently reported clinical trials in ALS have employed outcome measures that have not been truly validated. ALS is a disease whose ultimate outcome is death. Outcome measures such as muscle strength, function as detected by rating scales, or physiologic measures decline with disease progression, with faster rates of decline being correlated with survival. However, the effect on these measures of any therapeutic agent that alters survival has not been studied; thus their relative sensitivity compared to survival is unknown. This problem can be resolved only by a positive clinical trial in which multiple outcome measures are obtained and compared to survival.

Appendix

The NEALS Consortium members participating in this trial include:
Participating coordinators and clinical evaluators: C.L. Bagley, MA, T. Conrad, M. Chilton, MA, J. Taft, PA-C, SUNY Upstate Medical University; S. Hilgenberg,

L. Urbinelli, Massachusetts General Hospital; J. Florence, C. Harper, J. Schierbecker, Washington University; G.P. Hyde, S. Hinkle, B. Freiberg, Wake Forest University; D. Padgett, C. Foley-Schwartz, Mayo Clinic; J. Steele, B. Fitzgerald, University of Miami; J. Mass, University of California, San Francisco; T. Wheeler, D. Andrews-Hinders, K. Levin, A. Kloos, Cleveland Clinic; L. Hass, A. Michaels, Indiana University; C. Cook, T. Paylor, Y. Suh, MCP-Hahnemann University; P. Krusinski, S. Barsotti, University of Vermont; M. Del Bene, S. Hayes, Columbia Presbyterian Medical Center.

Steering Committee: J. Shefner (Principal Investigator), SUNY Upstate Medical University; M. Cudkowicz, D. Schoenfeld, Massachusetts General Hospital; J. Rothstein, Johns Hopkins University.

Safety Monitoring Committee: D. Schoenfeld (Chair), Massachusetts General Hospital; E. Logigian, University of Rochester; B. Jubelt, SUNY Upstate Medical University.

References

Andreassen, O.A., Dedeoglu, A., Klivenyi, P., Beal, M.F., *et al.* (2000). N-acetyl-L-cysteine improves survival and preserves motor performance in an animal model of familial amyotrophic lateral sclerosis [In Process Citation]. *NeuroReport*, 11, 2491–2493.

Bensimon, G., Lacomblez, L., & Meininger, V. (1994). A controlled trial of riluzole in amyotrophic lateral sclerosis. *New England Journal of Medicine*, 330, 585–591.

Beutner, G., Ruck, A., Riede, B., & Brdiczka, D. (1998). Complexes between porin, hexokinase, mitochondrial creatine kinase and adenylate translocator display properties of the permeability transition pore. Implication for regulation of permeability transition by the kinases. *Biochimica Et Biophysica Acta*, 1368, 7–18.

Brooks, B. (1994). El Escorial World Federation of Neurology criteria for the diagnosis of amyotrophic lateral scerosis. Subcommittee on Motor Neuron Diseases/Amyotrophic Lateral Sclerosis of the World Federation of Neurology Research Group on Neuromuscular Diseases and the El Escorial Clinical limits of amyotrophic lateral sclerosis. *Journal of the Neurological Sciences*, 124 (Suppl), 96–107.

Brown, W.F., Strong, M.J., & Snow, R. (1988). Methods for estimating numbers of motor units in biceps–brachialis muscles and losses of motor units with aging. *Muscle Nerve*, 11, 423–432.

Bruijn, L.I., Beal, M.F., Becher, M.W., Schulz, J.B., *et al.* (1997). Elevated free nitrotyrosine levels, but not protein-bound nitrotyrosine or hydroxyl radicals, throughout amyotrophic lateral sclerosis (ALS)-like disease implicate tyrosine nitration as an aberrant *in vivo* property of one familial ALS-linked superoxide dismutase 1 mutant. *Proceedings of the National Academy of Sciences, USA*, 94, 7606–7611.

Carter, G.T., Krivickas, L.S., Weydt, P., Weiss, M.D., *et al.* (2003). Drug therapy for amyotrophic lateral sclerosis: Where are we now?. *Idrugs*, 6, 147–153.

Cedarbaum, J.M., Stambler, N., Malta, E., Fuller, C., *et al.* (1999). The ALSFRS-R: a revised ALS functional rating scale that incorporates assessments of respiratory function. BDNF ALS Study Group (Phase III). *Journal of the Neurological Sciences*, 169, 13–21.

Chio, A., & Silani, V. (2001). Amyotrophic lateral sclerosis care in Italy: a nationwide study in neurological centers. *Journal of Neurological Sciences*, 191, 145–150.

Cudkowicz, M.E., Shefner, J.M., Schoenfeld, D.A., Brown, Jr., R.H., *et al.* (2003). A randomized, placebo-controlled trial of topiramate in amyotrophic lateral sclerosis. *Neurology*, 61, 456–464.

Dal Canto, M.C. (1995). Comparison of pathological alterations in ALS and a murine transgenic model: pathogenetic implications. *Clinical Neuroscience*, 3, 332–337.

Drachman, D.B., Frank, K., Dykes-Hoberg, M., Teismann, P., et al. (2002). Cyclo-oxygenase 2 inhibition protects motor neurons and prolongs survival in a transgenic mouse model of ALS. *Annals of Neurology*, 52, 771–778.

Eisen, A., & Weber, M. (1999). Treatment of amyotrophic lateral sclerosis. *Drugs Aging*, 14, 173–196.

Ferrante, R.J., Browne, S.E., Shinobu, L.A., Bowling, A.C., et al. (1997). Evidence of increased oxidative damage in both sporadic and familial amyotrophic lateral sclerosis. *Journal of Neurochemistry*, 69, 2064–2074.

Gredal, O., Werdelin, L., Bak, S., Christensen, P.B., et al. (1997). A clinical trial of dextromethorphan in amyotrophic lateral sclerosis. *Acta Neurologica Scandinavia*, 96, 8–13.

Groeneveld, G.J., Veldink, J.H., van der Tweel, I., Kalmijn, S., et al. (2003). A randomized sequential trial of creatine in amyotrophic lateral sclerosis. *Annals of Neurology*, 53, 437–445.

Group A-CTS. (1996). A double-blind placebo-controlled clinical trial of subcutaneous recombinant human ciliary neurotophic factor (rHCNTF) in amyotrophic lateral sclerosis. *Neurology*, 46, 1244–1249.

Gubbay, S.S., Kahana, E., Zilber, N., Cooper, G., et al. (1985). Amyotrophic lateral sclerosis. A study of its presentation and prognosis. *Journal of Neurology*, 232, 295–300.

Gurney, M.E., Cutting, F.B., Zhai, P., Doble, A., et al. (1996). Benefit of vitamin E, riluzole and gabapentin in a transgenic model of familial amyotrophic lateral sclerosis [see comments]. *Annals of Neurology*, 39, 147–157.

Gurney, M.E., Fleck, T.J., Himes, C.S., & Hall, E.D. (1998). Riluzole preserves motor function in a transgenic model of familial amyotrophic lateral sclerosis. *Neurology*, 50, 62–66.

Haverkamp, L.J., Appel, V., & Appel, S.H. (1995). Natural history of amyotrophic lateral sclerosis in a database population. Validation of a scoring system and a model for survival prediction. *Brain*, 118 (Pt 3), 707–719.

Hemmer, W., & Wallimann, T. (1993). Functional aspects of creatine kinase in brain. *Developmental Neuroscience*, 15, 249–260.

Hirano, A. (1991). Cytopathology in amyotrophic lateral sclerosis. *Advanced Neurology*, 56, 91–101.

Jablecki, C.K., Berry, C., & Leach, J. (1989). Survival prediction in amyotrophic lateral sclerosis. *Muscle Nerve*, 12, 833–841.

Julien, J.P., Couillard-Despres, S., & Meier, J. (1998). Transgenic mice in the study of ALS: the role of neurofilaments. *Brain Pathology*, 8, 759–769.

Julien, J.P., & Mushynski, W.E. (1998). Neurofilaments in health and disease. *Progress in Nucleic Acid Research and Molecular Biology*, 61, 1–23.

Klivenyi, P., Ferrante, R.J., Matthews, R.T., Bogdanov, M.B., et al. (1999). Neuro-protective effects of creatine in a transgenic animal model of amyotrophic lateral sclerosis. *Natural Medicine*, 5, 347–350.

Klivenyi, P., Kiaei, M., Gardian, G., Calingasan, N.Y., et al. (2004). Additive neuro-protective effects of creatine and cyclooxygenase 2 inhibitors in a transgenic mouse model of amyotrophic lateral sclerosis. *Journal of Neurochemistry*, 88, 576–582.

Kong, J., & Xu, Z. (1998). Massive mitochondrial degeneration in motor neurons triggers the onset of amyotrophic lateral sclerosis in mice expressing a mutant SOD1. *Journal of Neurosciences*, 18, 3241–3250.

Kurtzke, J. (1989). Risk factors in amyotrophic lateral sclerosis. *Advanced Neurology*, 56, 245–270.

Kurtzke, J., & Kurland, L. (1989). The epidemiology of neurologic disease. In: Joynt, R. (ed.), *Clinical Neurology*, Philadelphia, PA: Lippincott, pp. 1–43.

Lacomblez, L., Bensimon, G., Leigh, P., Guillett, P., et al. (1996). Dose-ranging study of riluzole in amyotrophic lateral sclerosis. *Lancet*, 347, 1428–1431.

Lai, E.C., Felice, K.J., Festoff, B.W., Gawel, M.J., *et al.* (1997). Effect of recombinant human insulin-like growth factor-I on progression of ALS. A placebo-controlled study. The North America ALS/IGF-I Study Group. *Neurology*, 49, 1621–1630.

Masui, Y., Mozai, T., & Kakehi, K. (1985). Functional and morphometric study of the liver in motor neuron disease. *Journal of Neurology*, 232, 15–19.

Miller, R.G., Moore, D.H., Gelinas, D.F., Dronsky, V., *et al.* (2001). Phase III randomized trial of gabapentin in patients with amyotrophic lateral sclerosis. *Neurology*, 56, 843–848.

Miller, R.G., Petajan, J.H., Bryan, W.W., Armon, C., *et al.* (1996). A placebo-controlled trial of recombinant human ciliary neurotrophic (rhCNTF) factor in amyotrophic lateral sclerosis. rhCNTF ALS Study Group. *Annals of Neurology*, 39, 256–260.

Mulder, D. (1982). Clinical Limits of Amyotrophic Lateral Sclerosis. In: Rowland, L.P. (ed.), Human Motor Neuron Diseases, New York: Raven Press, pp. 15–22.

Nakano, K., Hirayama, K., & Terai, K. (1987). Hepatic ultrastructural changes and liver dysfunction in amyotrophic lateral sclerosis. *Archieves Neurology*, 44, 103–106.

Ro, L.S., Lai, S.L., Chen, C.M., & Chen, S.T. (2003). Deleted 4977-bp mitochondrial DNA mutation is associated with sporadic amyotrophic lateral sclerosis: a hospital based case–control study. *Muscle Nerve*, 28, 737–743.

Robberecht, W. (2000). Oxidative stress in amyotrophic lateral sclerosis. *Journal of Neurology*, 247 (Suppl 1), I1–I6.

Rosen, D., Siddique, T., Patterson, D., Figlewicz, D., *et al.* (1993). Mutations in Cu/Zn superoxide dismutase gene are associated with familial amyotrophic lateral sclerosis. *Nature*, 362, 59–62.

Rothstein, J.D. (1996). Excitotoxicity hypothesis. *Neurology*, 47, S19–S25; discussion S26.

Rothstein, J.D., Dykes-Hoberg, M., Pardo, C.A., Bristol, L.A., *et al.* (1996). Knockout of glutamate transporters reveals a major role for astroglial transport in excitotoxicity and clearance of glutamate. *Neuron*, 16, 675–686.

Rothstein, J.D., Patel, S., Regan, M.R., Haenggeli, C., *et al.* (2005). Beta-lactam antibiotics offer neuroprotection by increasing glutamate transporter expression. *Nature*, 433, 73–77.

Rouleau, G.A., Clark, A.W., Rooke, K., Pramatarova, A., *et al.* (1996). SOD1 mutation is associated with accumulation of neurofilaments in amyotrophic lateral sclerosis. *Annals of Neurology*, 39, 128–131.

Rowland, L.P. (1994). Amyotrophic lateral sclerosis. *Current Opinion in Neurology*, 7, 310–315.

Sasaki, S., & Iwata, M. (1999). Ultrastructural change of synapses of Betz cells in patients with amyotrophic lateral sclerosis. *Neuroscience Letters*, 268, 29–32.

Schiefer, J., Landwehrmeyer, G.B., Luesse, H.G., Sprunken, A., *et al.* (2002). Riluzole prolongs survival time and alters nuclear inclusion formation in a transgenic mouse model of Huntington's disease. *Movement Disorders*, 17, 748–757.

Schinder, A., Olson, E., Spitzer, N., & Montal, M. (1996). Mitochondrial dysfunction is a primary event in glutamate neurotoxicity. *Journal of Neurosciences*, 16, 6125–6133.

Shefner, J.M. (1996). Amyotrophic lateral sclerosis. In: Samuels, M.A., & Feske, S. (eds.). Office Practice of Neurology, New York: Churchill Living Stone, pp. 474–479.

Shefner, J.M., Tyler, H.R., & Krarup, C. (1991). Abnormalities in the sensory action potential in patients with amyotrophic lateral sclerosis. *Muscle Nerve*, 14, 1242–1246.

Snow, R.J., Turnbull, J., da Silva, S., Jiang, F., *et al.* (2003). Creatine supplementation and riluzole treatment provide similar beneficial effects in copper, zinc superoxide dismutase (G93A) transgenic mice. *Neuroscience*, 119, 661–667.

Traynor, B., Zhang, H., Shefner, J., Schoenfeld, D., *et al.* (2004). Functional outcome measures as clinical trial endpoints in Amyotrophic Lateral Sclerosis. *Neurology*, 63, 1933–1935.

Trotti, D., Rolfs, A., Danbolt, N.C., Brown, Jr., R.H., *et al.* (1999). SOD1 mutants linked to amyotrophic lateral sclerosis selectively inactivate a glial glutamate transporter [published erratum appears in *Natural Neurosciences*, 2(9), 848]. *Natural Neurosciences*, 2, 427–433.

White, R., & Reynolds, I. (1996). Mitochondrial depolarization in glutamate-stimulated neurons: an early signal specific to excitotoxin exposure. *Journal of Neurosciences*, 16, 5688–5697.

Wong, P.C., Pardo, C.A., Borchelt, D.R., Lee, M.K., *et al.* (1995). An adverse property of a familial ALS-linked SOD1 mutation causes motor neuron disease characterized by vacuolar degeneration of mitochondria. *Neuron*, 14, 1105–1116.

Zhang, W., Narayanan, M., & Friedlander, R.M. (2003). Additive neuroprotective effects of minocycline with creatine in a mouse model of ALS. *Annals of Neurology*, 53, 267–270.

Progress in Neurotherapeutics and Neuropsychopharmacology, 1:1, 91–104 © 2006 Cambridge University Press
DOI: 10.1017/S1748232105000091   Printed in the United Kingdom

AVP-923 as a Novel Treatment for Pseudobulbar Affect in ALS

Laura E. Pope
Clinical and Regulatory Affairs, Avanir Pharmaceuticals, San Diego, CA 92121, USA;
Email: LPope@avanir.com

Key words: Pseudobulbar palsy; pathologic laughing; pathologic crying; dextromethorphan; quinidine; amyotrophic lateral sclerosis; multiple sclerosis; clinical trial; neurotherapeutics.

Introduction and Overview

Pseudobulbar affect (PBA) is a neurologic condition characterized by the disinhibition or loss of control of the motor expression of emotion (Wilson, 1924). Hallmark symptoms of PBA are uncontrollable crying and/or laughing that is out of context with the social setting (Arciniegas & Topkoff, 2000; Dark *et al.*, 1996). The condition can be severe, unremitting, and persistent (Dark *et al.*, 1996). PBA occurs secondary to neurologic diseases or injuries including amyotrophic lateral sclerosis (ALS) (Gallagher, 1989), multiple sclerosis (MS) (Feinstein *et al.*, 1997), stroke (House *et al.*, 1989), traumatic brain injury (Zeilig *et al.*, 1996), Parkinson's disease (Kaschka *et al.*, 2001), and dementia, including Alzheimer's disease (Starkstein *et al.*, 1995). Other terms used to refer to PBA include pathologic laughing and crying (PLC), emotional lability (EL), and emotional incontinence (Dark *et al.*, 1996).

PBA is caused by structural damage to the brain (Dark *et al.*, 1996), possibly resulting from excitotoxic mechanisms underlying the associated neurologic disorder (Mattson, 2003). The end result is disconnection of the regions of the brain that regulate the motor expression of emotion. Under normal conditions, cortical regions (prefrontal, frontal, temporal, and motor), as well as subcortical limbic structures, send modulated signals to the cerebellum and brainstem to coordinate appropriate displays of emotion (Parvizi *et al.*, 2001; Arciniegas & Topkoff, 2000; Mega *et al.*, 1997; Wilson, 1924). It is hypothesized that abnormally increased excitatory, glutamatergic signaling causes the damage underlying a variety of

----

Correspondence should be addressed to: Laura E. Pope, PhD, Clinical and Regulatory Affairs, Avanir Pharmaceuticals, 11388 Sorrento Valley Road, Suite 200, San Diego, CA 92121, USA. Ph: +858 622 5207; Fax: +858 622 4607; Email: LPope@avanir.com.

neurologic disease and injury states (Mattson, 2003; Bittigau & Ikonomidou, 1997; Greenamyre, 1986), including a role in all those listed above that are linked with PBA (Mattson, 2003; Matute *et al.*, 2001; Bittigau & Ikonomidou, 1997). If excitotoxic damage impacts brain networks that mediate emotional expression, the result may be involuntary displays of affect such as crying and/or laughing (Arciniegas & Topkoff, 2000). In ALS and MS, PBA commonly occurs with corticobulbar degeneration that effectively releases cortical inhibition of brainstem centers that organize laughing/crying responses (Feinstein *et al.*, 1997; Caroscio *et al.*, 1987; Black, 1982; Lieberman & Benson, 1977; Wilson, 1924).

A novel agent in development to treat PBA, AVP-923, is believed to exert its therapeutic effects via anti-excitatory actions. The active component of AVP-923 reduces glutamatergic responses (Maurice *et al.*, 2001; Maurice & Lockhart, 1997; Annels *et al.*, 1991), and has been shown to preferentially bind in brain regions (Musacchio *et al.*, 1989; Tortella *et al.*, 1989) thought to be involved in the control of emotional displays (Parvizi *et al.*, 2001; Wilson, 1924).

Rationale (Purpose of Trial)

Up to 50% of ALS patients exhibit PBA, and it is more prevalent in those with bulbar symptoms (Gallagher, 1989). PBA can be profoundly disabling in social and occupational settings. It is distressful and embarrassing to both patients and their caregivers (Arciniegas & Topkoff, 2000; Shaibani *et al.*, 1994). There are currently no drugs approved by the US Food and Drug Administration (US FDA) for the treatment of PBA. This chapter describes the results of a multicenter, controlled trial designed to evaluate the efficacy, safety, and tolerability of AVP-923 for the treatment of PBA in ALS (Brooks *et al.*, 2004).

Agent: AVP-923

AVP-923 is a capsule containing a fixed combination of dextromethorphan hydrobromide (DM, 30 mg) and quinidine sulfate (Q, 30 mg). AVP-923 was administered twice daily (every 12 h, Q12H) in clinical studies for PBA.

Dextromethorphan Hydrobromide

The mechanism by which AVP-923 relieves PBA is unknown. However, based on available evidence, its therapeutic effect may result from a reduction of excitatory, glutamatergic neurotransmission in brain networks regulating emotional expression. The active component of AVP-923 is DM, a sigma-1 receptor agonist (Maurice *et al.*, 2001; Klein & Musacchio, 1989) and an uncompetitive *N*-methyl-D-aspartate

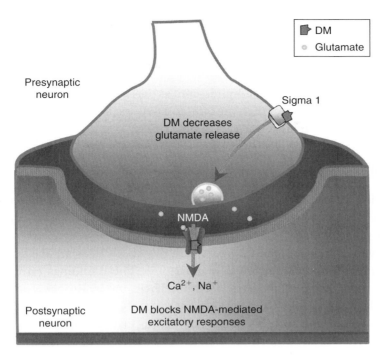

Fig. 1.
DM acts as a sigma-1 receptor agonist and an uncompetitive NMDA receptor antagonist to decrease excitatory, glutamatergic signaling. Ca^{2+}: calcium; Na^+: sodium.

(NMDA) receptor antagonist (Ebert *et al.*, 1998; Maurice & Lockhart, 1997; Tortella *et al.*, 1989) (Figure 1). Sigma receptors modulate neurotransmitter release (Maurice & Lockhart, 1997), and DM has been shown to decrease glutamate release *in vitro* (Annels *et al.*, 1991). DM also blocks NMDA responses to glutamate (Maurice & Lockhart, 1997). Sigma-1 sites are particularly concentrated in the brainstem and cerebellum (Maurice *et al.*, 2001; Debonnel & de Montigny, 1996), regions believed to play a role in emotional motor responses (Parvizi *et al.*, 2001; Wilson, 1924).

Quinidine Sulfate

A low dose of Q (30 mg) serves to maximally inhibit the rapid first-pass metabolism of DM, thereby increasing its systemic availability and potential therapeutic utility (Pope *et al.*, 2004; Zhang *et al.*, 1992). DM is extensively metabolized in about 90% of the population (Droll *et al.*, 1998) by the hepatic cytochrome P450 2D6 enzyme (CYP2D6), which catalyzes the *O*-demethylation of DM to its main metabolite dextrorphan (DX). Blood levels of DM increase linearly with DM dose following co-administration with Q, but are undetectable in most patients given DM alone, even at high doses (Zhang *et al.*, 1992). Thus, treatment with the fixed combination of DM plus Q allows the attainment of predictable and sustainable blood levels of DM that have a greater likelihood of reaching neuronal targets (Pope *et al.*, 2004).

Importantly, the daily Q dose administered as part of AVP-923 therapy (30 mg Q12H) is 10 to 25 times lower than the 600- to 1600-mg daily dose routinely used to treat cardiac arrhythmias (Grace & Camm, 1998).

Past Clinical Experience

A combination of DM (30 mg) and Q (75 mg) given twice daily to ALS patients was initially found to suppress PBA in a double-blind, placebo-controlled crossover study ($p < 0.001$). This trial included 12 ALS patients, and treatment lasted for 2 weeks with drug and 2 weeks with placebo. PBA was assessed with a validated self-report measure (Smith *et al.*, 1995). These findings provided the rationale for the Phase III clinical trial described here and by Brooks *et al.* (2004).

Phase I clinical studies in healthy subjects ($N = 111$) determined the lowest dose of Q needed to sufficiently increase DM bioavailability. Varying doses of Q were given twice daily with DM for 7 days. The elevation in DM plasma levels appeared approximately linear up to 30 mg of Q and then plateaued, indicating that this low dose of Q maximally suppressed *O*-demethylation of DM at steady state (Pope *et al.*, 2004). These findings provided the basis for the combination of fixed doses selected for AVP-923.

Clinical Trial

This multicenter, double-blind, controlled study of the treatment of PBA in ALS had a parallel, three-arm design (Figure 2). Subjects were randomized by center (17 centers) to receive AVP-923 (30 mg DM plus 30 mg Q), DM (30 mg) alone, or Q (30 mg) alone, with twice as many subjects receiving AVP-923 as either DM or Q (2 : 1 : 1 ratio). Capsules were taken orally twice daily (approximately Q12H) for 28 days.

Subjects

Patients were enrolled between January 2001 and March 2002, and all completed treatment by April 30, 2002. Inclusion criteria included (1) a diagnosis of probable or definite ALS according to the World Federation of Neurology that was made more than 2 months prior to study and (2) a history of PBA with a cut-off score of ⩾13 on the Center for Neurologic Study Liability Scale (CNS-LS) (described below). The main exclusion criteria were abnormal electrocardiographs (ECGs), major concurrent illnesses, and a history of major psychiatric disturbance or

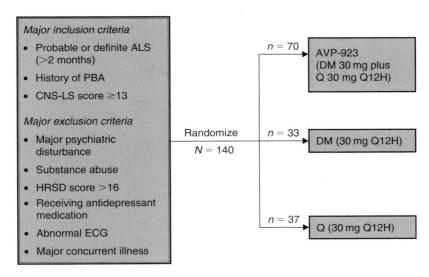

Fig. 2.
Clinical trial parallel, three-arm design and subject disposition.

substance abuse. Furthermore, patients with a Hamilton Rating Scale for Depression (HRSD) score >16 (moderate depression) or those being treated with anti-depressants were excluded (Figure 2).

The intention-to-treat (ITT) population was prospectively defined as subjects who were not poor metabolizers of DM, because theoretically Q would not be required for efficacy in poor metabolizers since DM levels are naturally elevated. The ITT population was analyzed for efficacy and included 65 AVP-923 patients, 30 DM patients, and 34 Q patients. For the primary efficacy endpoint, four AVP-923 subjects completed only day 1 of testing, resulting in an evaluable ITT population of 61. Safety was assessed in all randomized subjects ($N = 140$; Figure 2).

The ITT cohort included 80 men and 49 women. The mean age was about 55 years (range of 33–82 years), and about 88% of patients were white. There were no significant demographic differences between treatment groups.

Methods

INSTRUMENTS/MEASURES

The CNS-LS was used to measure PBA. This seven-item self-administered scale has been validated in a large population of ALS patients (Moore *et al.*, 1997). Two 10-cm Visual Analog Scales (VASs) were used to assess quality of life (QOL) and quality of relationships (QOR) (Huskisson, 1974). The VASs asked the patient to, "Please place a slash (/not X) on the scale below to indicate how much uncontrollable laughter, tearfulness, or anger has affected the overall quality of your life (*or overall quality of your relationships with others*) during the past week" on 10-cm lines anchored with "Not at all" on the left and "Continuously" on the right. The HRSD was used to evaluate depression. CYP2D6 genotyping was performed to determine extensive and poor metabolizer phenotypes. Blood samples were taken on day 29 within 8 h following the last dose to measure concentrations of DM, its metabolite DX, and Q.

PRIMARY AND SECONDARY OUTCOMES

The primary efficacy variable was the change from baseline in CNS-LS score. Secondary efficacy endpoints were (1) the number of laughing and/or crying episodes per week recorded in patient diaries, (2) change from baseline in QOL scores, and (3) change from baseline in QOR scores.

ANALYSIS

Patients were assessed prior to dosing on day 1 (baseline), and on days 15 and 29. All efficacy variables involving a change were determined as the baseline score subtracted from the mean of the scores on days 15 and 29. Changes in CNS-LS, QOL, and QOR were determined using linear regression models and adjusted for baseline score and study center. Episode counts and the relationship between episode rates and CNS-LS were evaluated using a negative binomial regression model to control for site differences and high individual variability. Secondary efficacy variables were also combined and analyzed with the O'Brien rank sum method (O'Brien, 1984) to account for multiple comparisons. Adverse events (AEs) were compared using the Fisher's exact test. All p-values reported are two-sided. An α-value of 0.05 was used for significance.

Results

EFFICACY

Inhibition of DM Metabolism by Q. There was a significant pharmacokinetic/ pharmacodynamic correlation between increased DM plasma levels and effect (improvement on CNS-LS). The mean DM plasma concentration was 18-fold higher in the AVP-923 group (96.4 ± 46.7 ng/ml, mean ± SD, $n = 35$) than in the DM group (5.2 ± 5.0 ng/ml, $n = 23$; $p < 0.0001$). The mean concentration of DX, the major metabolite of DM, was 3.3-fold lower in the AVP-923 group (89.5 ± 52.3 ng/ml) than in the DM group (295.9 ± 143.2 ng/ml; $p < 0.0001$). Only pharmacokinetic samples drawn within 8 h after the last dose were included in the bioanalysis.

Analysis of Q revealed a median level of 150 ng/ml (range, <LOQ, the limit of quantitation to 2210 ng/ml) in the AVP-923 group and a median level of 80 ng/ml (range, <LOQ to 200 ng/ml) in the Q group. Q levels with this dose regimen often dip below the LOQ of 0.05 μg/ml during the 8-h collection window (Pope *et al.*, 2004).

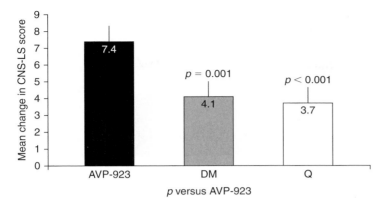

Fig. 3.
Treatment with AVP-923 (DM plus Q) resulted in about a 3.5-point greater improvement on the CNS-LS than treatment with DM or Q alone. Values plotted are least-squares mean ± SE; adjusting for baseline levels and center effects.

Improvement in CNS-LS Score.   As prospectively defined in the statistical analysis plan, the difference in mean CNS-LS improvement was adjusted for two important, prospectively defined covariates: baseline CNS-LS score and study center. The average adjusted decrease of CNS-LS in the AVP-923 group was 3.29 points greater than in the DM group ($p = 0.001$) and 3.71 points greater than in the Q group ($p < 0.001$) (Figure 3).

Decreased Laughing/Crying Episodes.   The mean number of laughing or crying episodes per week recorded in patient diaries was 1.9 times lower in the AVP-923 group than in the DM group ($p = 0.004$) and 2.1 times lower than in the Q group ($p < 0.001$). Corresponding ratios for crying and laughing were similar. Significantly more patients in the AVP-923 group (52%) were symptom-free over the last 2 weeks of the study compared to the DM (23%) and Q (12%) groups ($p < 0.001$). The median number of episode-free days was 23 for the AVP-923 group compared to 6 and 11 days for the DM and Q groups, respectively ($p = 0.007$).

Improved QOL and QOR.   The adjusted mean changes from baseline in VAS scores for QOL and QOR were greater in the AVP-923 group compared to both active control groups at all time points examined (Figure 4). These results indicate improved QOL and QOR. Similar results are observed when the day 15 and 29 results were analyzed individually rather than as an average (not shown) indicating an effect as early as day 15 of treatment.

Simultaneous Analysis of Secondary Efficacy Variables.   To account for multiple comparisons, all secondary efficacy variables were combined and evaluated using

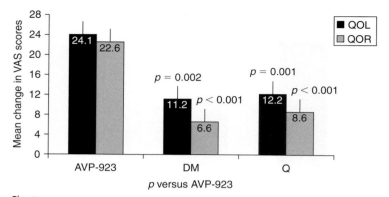

Fig. 4.
Treatment with AVP-923 (DM plus Q) resulted in significantly greater improvements on the VAS scores for QOL and QOR than treatment with DM or Q alone. Values plotted are least-squares mean ± SE; adjusting for baseline levels and center effects.

the non-parametric method of O'Brien (1984). This analysis demonstrated that AVP-923 subjects had reduced episode rates and improved QOL and QOR scores relative to subjects treated with DM ($p = 0.004$) or Q ($p < 0.001$).

Sensitivity Analyses.   The substantial findings, including significance, do not change when all randomized patients ($N = 140$) are included in the analysis.

SAFETY AND TOLERABILITY

AVP-923 is generally safe and well tolerated. Most AEs were mild or moderate. There were no treatment-related serious AEs. Treatment-related discontinuations included 24% ($n = 17$) of AVP-923, 6% ($n = 2$) of DM, and 87% ($n = 3$) of Q patients. Most AEs (92%) in subjects who discontinued were mild or moderate, and the effects were reversible. Discontinuations occurred early in the trial, and more than 90% of subjects in the AVP-923 group who tolerated the drug for the first 5 days of dosing completed the 28-day treatment. This observation, along with findings from a recent open-label study of AVP-923 in diabetic neuropathy (Thisted, Pope, *et al.*, unpublished data), suggests that better tolerability may be obtained by starting with once a day dosing. Overall, improved QOL and QOR scores suggests that the benefit from treatment with AVP-923 outweighs the discomfort caused by AEs.

AEs reported in ⩾5% of patients are listed in Table 1. Commonly experienced AEs that occurred significantly more frequently with study drug versus active control treatments included nausea, dizziness, and somnolence. These are established AEs of DM, and since Q enhances DM bioavailability, the increased incidence of these effects with AVP-923 was predicted. Gastrointestinal complaints were also as expected based on previous use of DM and Q, and many AEs appeared specific to ALS patients (e.g. muscle cramps, muscle spasms, and weakness).

Table 1. **Percentage of Patients (⩾5% in Any Treatment Group) with AEs: Safety Population (*N* = 140)**

AE	AVP-923 (*N* = 70)	DM (*N* = 33)	Q (*N* = 37)
Anorexia	5.7	3.0	0.0
Anxiety NEC	4.3	0.0	8.1
Arthralgia	2.9	9.1	5.4
Constipation	7.1	6.1	0.0
Confusion	1.4	6.1	0.0
Diarrhea NOS	15.7	21.2	10.8
Dizziness (excluding vertigo)[a]	20.0	15.2	2.7
Dyspnea NOS	2.9	0.0	8.1
Edema lower limb	0.0	3.0	5.4
Fall	8.6	6.1	0.0
Fatigue	18.6	9.1	10.8
Flatulence	1.4	6.1	0.0
Headache NOS	15.7	12.1	10.8
Hypertonia	7.1	0.0	2.7
Joint stiffness	10.0	0.0	2.7
Localized infection	0.0	0.0	5.4
Loose stools[a]	0.0	9.1	0.0
Muscle cramps	7.1	6.1	2.7
Muscle spasms	2.9	6.1	0.0
Nasopharyngitis	1.4	9.1	2.7
Nausea[a]	32.9	6.1	8.1
Pruritus NOS	0.0	0.0	5.4
Sinus congestion	2.9	6.1	2.7
Sleep disorder NOS	0.0	0.0	5.4
Somnolence[a]	12.9	3.0	0.0
Sweating increased	5.7	0.0	2.7
Upper respiratory tract infection NOS	4.3	3.0	5.4
Vomiting NOS	5.7	0.0	0.0
Weakness	5.7	3.0	10.8

AEs were reported by 89% of AVP-923, 70% of DM, and 65% of Q patients.
NEC: not elsewhere classified; NOS: not otherwise specified; AVP-923: fixed combination of DM plus Q.
[a] Number reported significantly different between groups.

There was no evidence for cardiac effects of Q, and bioanalytical results demonstrated very low exposure levels. Mean quinidine levels in the blood measured at least 10 times lower than the therapeutic anti-arrhythmia level, and QT_c intervals (and all other ECG parameters evaluated) were not clinically significantly affected.

Poor Metabolizers.   Poor metabolizers of DM, constitute ≤7% of the population (Droll *et al.*, 1998). In these individuals, the DM/Q combination (AVP-923) does not raise DM levels above levels attained with DM-only treatment (Schadel *et al.*, 1995). Following AVP-923 administration, exposure to DM is similar in poor and extensive metabolizers (Pope *et al.*, 2004). Therefore AVP-923 should be equally therapeutic in poor and extensive metabolizers with a similar safety profile.

Drug Interactions.   Since Q inhibits CYP2D6, caution must be exercised whenever prescribing AVP-923 together with drugs extensively metabolized by CYP2D6 (e.g. most polycyclic antidepressants): http://www.watsonpharm.com. Furthermore, there is evidence that DM can modulate serotonin (5-hydroxytryptamine, 5-HT) release (Kamei *et al.*, 1992), and due to the potential to develop 5-HT syndrome (Gillman, 2005), DM is contraindicated in patients receiving monoamine oxidase inhibitors (MAOIs; http://www.mc.uky.edu/pharmacy/DIC/DDI/DextromethorphanMAOIDDI.htm).

Unique Aspects of Trial

AVP-923 is a novel treatment option for PBA in ALS and is the first agent proven effective in a large, controlled clinical trial. This uniquely proportioned combination of DM and Q is significantly more effective than either of its components alone. Although DM is the active ingredient, the low dose of Q is needed to elevate DM levels to the therapeutic range. Notably, AVP-923 is the first treatment demonstrated to improve QOL in the ALS population. Although antidepressants have been used off-label to treat PBA with some success (discussed below) (Nahas *et al.*, 1998; Mukand *et al.*, 1996; Robinson *et al.*, 1993; Schiffer *et al.*, 1985), AVP-923 provides a distinct and unique therapeutic mechanism of action. DM may exert a specific action on brain regions (Musacchio *et al.*, 1989; Tortella *et al.*, 1989) implicated in emotional expression (Parvizi *et al.*, 2001; Wilson, 1924). Thus AVP-923 offers a potentially more selective approach to the treatment of PBA (Schiffer & Pope, 2005).

Conclusions

AVP-923 effectively and safely palliates PBA in ALS, and is significantly more effective than either of its components (DM and Q). Marked (approximately 2-fold) improvement was indicated by the CNS-LS, a validated self-assessment scale, and by a more than 40% decrease in laughing/crying episode rates compared to control groups. More than half of AVP-923 patients, and significantly more than those treated with DM or Q alone, were symptom-free over the last 2 weeks of the study. Overall benefits of treatment were further reflected in 2-fold or greater enhancements in QOL and QOR.

Influence on the Field

A multicenter, double-blind, placebo-controlled trial was recently conducted to assess the efficacy and safety of AVP-923 in the treatment of PBA associated with MS (Panitch *et al.*, 2005). Efficacy variables were similar to those in the ALS study. AVP-923 was administered for 3 months and resulted in marked improvements on all measures, with a low incidence of treatment-related AEs. Treatment effects were observed as early as the first week.

An ongoing open-label trial is being conducted to assess the safety of chronic exposure (at least 6 months) to AVP-923 in patients with PBA associated with various neurologic disorders including ALS, MS, stroke, Alzheimer's disease, Parkinson's disease, and traumatic brain injury. There is at least one case study report of palliation of PBA with AVP-923 in an Alzheimer's patient participating in this trial (Richter, 2005).

The clinical findings in the ALS population, along with these recent results showing efficacy of AVP-923 for the treatment of PBA in MS, support the idea that the neurochemical pathology underlying PBA may be similar across the various neurologic disorders with which it is associated (Shaibani *et al.*, 1994; Robinson *et al.*, 1993; Brooks *et al.*, 2004).

A New Drug Application (NDA) for AVP-923 or Neurodex™ for the treatment of PBA is in preparation for submission to the US FDA.

Translation to Clinical Practice

Currently there is no approved therapy with an indication for PBA. Off-label use of antidepressants has yielded only partial success, and may be limited by treatment-related AEs. Antidepressant use for PBA is supported by positive results from small comparative trials with tricyclics (TCAs) (Robinson *et al.*, 1993; Schiffer *et al.*, 1985) and selective serotonin reuptake inhibitors (SSRIs) (Burns *et al.*, 1999; Müller *et al.*, 1999; Andersen *et al.*, 1993). However, not all PBA patients respond to antidepressant treatment (Schiffer *et al.*, 1985), and none of these agents have been proven effective in large, well-controlled trials using a validated measurement instrument (Arciniegas & Topkoff, 2000). Moreover, while up to 50% of ALS patients suffer from PBA (Gallagher, 1989), only 11–22% of ALS patients are depressed (Ganzini *et al.*, 1999; Houpt *et al.*, 1977). Patients in this study were not depressed, as evidenced by mean HRSD scores of <6 at baseline and the end of treatment (a score of 16 is equal to "moderate" depression). This underscores the clear distinction between depression and PBA (Smith *et al.*, 2003; Robinson *et al.*, 1993). Finally, TCAs are associated with a high incidence of AEs, including anticholinergic effects (e.g. memory deficits) (Baldessarini, 1985), that are particularly problematic in the elderly. As a result, many patients with even severe PBA remain untreated at present and there is a need for new therapeutic options (Dark *et al.*, 1996; Schiffer & Pope, 2005).

AVP-923 holds the promise of becoming the first, proven effective therapy for PBA associated with neurologic disease or injury if approved by FDA. AEs are mostly mild or moderate. To increase tolerability, patients may receive once daily dosing for the first week of therapy, followed by twice daily dosing. Long-term use of AVP-923 may be necessary, and its safety is supported by interim results from the ongoing open-label study in which patients are being treated for at least 6 months.

Summary of Treatment Recommendations for PBA

AVP-923 effectively and safely palliates PBA in ALS, as demonstrated in this Phase III clinical trial. It is the first agent in development specifically for the treatment of PBA.

References

Andersen, G., Vestergaard, K., & Riis, J.O. (1993). Citalopram for post-stroke pathological crying. *Lancet*, 342, 837–839.

Annels, S.J., Ellis, Y., & Davies, J.A. (1991). Non-opioid antitussives inhibit endogenous glutamate release from rabbit hippocampal slices. *Brain Research*, 564, 341–343.

Arciniegas, D.B., & Topkoff, J. (2000). The neuropsychiatry of pathologic affect: an approach to evaluation and treatment. *Seminars in Clinical Neuropsychiatry*, 5, 290–306.

Baldessarini, R.J. (1985). Drugs and the treatment of psychiatric disorder. In: Gilman, A.G., Goodman, L.S., Rall, T.W., & Mujrad, F. (eds.), *The Pharmacologic Basis of Therapeutics* (7th ed.). New York: MacMillan, pp. 387–415.

Bittigau, P., & Ikonomidou, C. (1997). Glutamate in neurologic diseases. *Journal of Child Neurology*, 12, 471–485.

Black, D.W. (1982). Pathological laughter: a review of the literature. *Journal of Nervous and Mental Disease*, 170, 67–71.

Brooks, B.R., Thisted, R.A., Appel, S.H., Bradley, W.G., Olney, R.K., Berg, J.E., Pope, L.E., & Smith, R.A. (2004). Treatment of pseudobulbar affect in ALS with dextromethorphan/quinidine. A randomized trial. *Neurology*, 63, 1364–1370.

Burns, A., Russell, E., Stratton-Powell, H., Tyrell, P., O'Neill, P., & Baldwin, R. (1999). Sertraline in stroke-associated lability of mood. *International Journal of Geriatric Psychiatry*, 14, 681–685.

Caroscio, J.T., Mulvihill, M.N., Sterling, R., & Abrams, B. (1987). Amyotrophic lateral sclerosis. *Neurologic Clinics*, 5, 1–8.

Dark, F.L., McGrath, J.J., & Ron, M.A. (1996). Pathological laughing and crying. *Australian and New Zealand Journal of Psychiatry*, 30, 472–479.

Debonnel, G., & de Montigny, C. (1996). Modulation of NMDA and dopaminergic neurotransmissions by sigma ligands: possible implications for the treatment of psychiatric disorders. *Life Sciences*, 58, 721–734.

Droll, K., Bruce-Mensah, K., Otton, S.V., Gaedigk, A., Sellers, E.M., & Tyndale, R.F. (1998). Comparison of three CYP2D6 probe substrates and genotype in Ghanaians, Chinese and Caucasians. *Pharmacogenetics*, 8, 325–333.

Ebert, B., Thorkildsen, C., Andersen, S., Christrup, L.L., & Hjeds, H. (1998). Opioid analgesics as noncompetitive N-methyl-D-aspartate (NMDA) antagonists. *Biochemical Pharmacology*, 56, 553–559.

Feinstein, A., Feinstein, K., Gray, T., & O'Connor, P. (1997). Prevalence and neurobehavioral correlates of pathological laughing and crying in multiple sclerosis. *Archives of Neurology*, 54, 1116–1121.

Gallagher, J.P. (1989). Pathologic laughter and crying in ALS: a search for their origin. *Acta Neurologica Scandinavica*, 80, 114–117.

Ganzini, L., Johnston, W.S., & Hoffman, W.F. (1999). Correlates of suffering in amyotrophic lateral sclerosis. *Neurology*, 52, 1434–1440.

Gillman, P.K. (2005). Monoamine oxidase inhibitors, opioid analgesics and serotonin toxicity. *British Journal of Anaesthesia*, 95, 434–441.

Grace, A.A., & Camm, A.J. (1998). Quinidine. *New England Journal of Medicine*, 338, 35–45.

Greenamyre, J.T. (1986). The role of glutamate in neurotransmission and in neurologic disease. *Archives of Neurology*, 43, 1058–1063.

Houpt, J.L., Gould, B.S., & Norris, F.H.J. (1977). Psychological characteristics of patients with amyotrophic lateral sclerosis (ALS). *Psychosomatic Medicine*, 39, 299–303.

House, A., Dennis, M., Molyneux, A., Warlow, C., & Hawton, K. (1989). Emotionalism after stroke. *British Medical Journal*, 298, 991–994.

Kamei, J., Mori, T., Igarashi, H., & Kasuya, Y. (1992). Serotonin release in nucleus of the solitary tract and its modulation by antitussive drugs. *Research Communications in Chemical Pathology and Pharmacology*, 76, 371–374.

Kaschka, W.P., Meyer, A., Schier, K.R., & Fröscher, W. (2001). Treatment of pathological crying with citalopram. *Pharmacopsychiatry*, 34, 254–258.

Klein, M., & Musacchio, J.M. (1989). High affinity dextromethorphan binding sites in guinea pig brain. Effect of sigma ligands and other agents. *Journal of Pharmacology and Experimental Therapeutics*, 251, 207–215.

Lieberman, A., & Benson, F. (1977). Control of emotional expression in pseudobulbar palsy. *Archives of Neurology*, 34, 717–719.

Mattson, M.P. (2003). Excitotoxic and excitoprotective mechanisms: abundant targets for the prevention and treatment of neurodegenerative disorders. *Neuromolecular Medicine*, 3, 65–94.

Matute, C., Alberdi, E., Domercq, M., Perez-Cerda, F., Perez-Samartin, A., & Sanchez-Gomez, M.V. (2001). The link between excitotoxic oligodendroglial death and demyelinating diseases. *Trends in Neurosciences*, 24, 224–230.

Maurice, T., & Lockhart, B.P. (1997). Neuroprotective and anti-amnesic potentials of sigma (σ) receptor ligands. *Progress in Neuropsychopharmacology and Biological Psychiatry*, 21, 69–102.

Maurice, T., Urani, A., Phan, V.L., & Romieu, P. (2001). The interaction between neuroactive steroids and the sigma1 receptor function: behavioral consequences and therapeutic opportunities. *Brain Research Reviews*, 37, 116–132.

Mega, M.S., Cummings, J.L., Salloway, S., & Malloy, P. (1997). The limbic system: an anatomic, phylogenetic, and clinical perspective. In: Salloway, S., Malloy, P., & Cummings, J.L. (eds.), *The Neuropsychiatry of Limbic and Subcortical Disorders*. Washington, DC: American Psychiatric Press, Inc., pp. 3–18.

Moore, S.R., Gresham, L.S., Bromberg, M.B., Kasarkis, E.J., & Smith, R.A. (1997). A self report measure of affective lability. *Journal of Neurology Neurosurgery and Psychiatry*, 63, 89–93.

Mukand, J., Kaplan, M., Senno, R.G., & Bishop, D.S. (1996). Pathological crying and laughing: treatment with sertraline. *Archives of Physical Medicine and Rehabilitation*, 77, 1309–1311.

Müller, U., Murai, T., Bauer-Wittmund, T., & von Cramon, D.Y. (1999). Paroxetine versus citalopram treatment of pathological crying after brain injury. *Brain Injury*, 13, 805–811.

Musacchio, J.M., Klein, M., & Canoll, P.D. (1989). Dextromethorphan and sigma ligands: common sites but diverse effects. *Life Sciences*, 45, 1721–1732.

Nahas, Z., Arlinghaus, K.A., Kotrla, K.J., Clearman, R.R., & George, M.S. (1998). Rapid response of emotional incontinence to selective serotonin reuptake inhibitors. *Journal of Neuropsychiatry and Clinical Neurosciences*, 10, 453–455.

O'Brien, P.C. (1984). Procedures for comparing samples with multiple endpoints. *Biometrics*, 40, 1079–1087.

Panitch, H., Thisted, R.A., Pope, L.E., & Berg, J.E. (2005). A double-blind, placebo-controlled, multicenter study to assess the safety and efficacy of AVP-923 (dextromethorphan/quinidine) in the treatment of pseudobulbar affect in patients with multiple sclerosis. *American Academy of Neurology 57th Annual Meeting*, Miami Beach, Florida, S46.001.

Parvizi, J., Anderson, S.W., Martin, C.O., Damasio, H., & Damasio, A.R. (2001). Pathological laughter and crying/a link to the cerebellum. *Brain*, 124, 1708–1719.

Pope, L.E., Khalil, M.H., Berg, J.E., Stiles, M., Yakatan, G.J., & Sellers, E.M. (2004). Pharmacokinetics of dextromethorphan after single or multiple dosing in combination with quinidine in extensive and poor metabolizers. *Journal of Clinical Pharmacology*, 44, 1132–1142.

Robinson, R.G., Parikh, R.M., Lipsey, J.R., Starkstein, S.E., & Price, T.R. (1993). Pathological laughing and crying following stroke: validation of a measurement scale and a double-blind treatment study. *American Journal of Psychiatry*, 150, 286–293.

Richter, R.W. (2005). Pseudobulbar affect in dementia improved under treatment with dextromethorphan/quinidine (AVP-923). *American Association for Geriatric Psychiatry Meeting*, San Diego, California.

Schadel, M., Wu, D., Otton, S.V., Kalow, W., & Sellers, E.M. (1995). Pharmacokinetics of dextromethorphan and metabolites in humans: influence of the CYP2D6 phenotype and quinidine inhibition. *Journal of Clinical Psychopharmacology*, 15, 263–269.

Schiffer, R., & Pope, L.E. (2005). Review of pseudobulbar affect including a novel and new potential therapy. *Journal of Neuropsychiatry and Clinical Neurosciences*, 17, 447–454.

Schiffer, R.B., Herndon, R.M., & Rudick, R.A. (1985). Treatment of pathologic laughing and weeping with amitriptyline. *New England Journal of Medicine*, 312, 1480–1482.

Shaibani, A.T., Sabbagh, M.N., & Doody, R. (1994). Laughter and crying in neurologic disorders. *Neuropsychiatry*, 7, 243–250.

Smith, R., Berg, J., Pope, L., & Thisted, R. (2003). Distinguishing affective disorders in amyotrophic lateral sclerosis. *14th International Symposium on ALS/MND*, Milan, Italy.

Smith, R.A., Moore, S.R., Gresham, L.S., Manley, P.E., & Licht, J.M. (1995). The treatment of affective lability in ALS patients with dextromethorphan. *Neurology*, 45, A330.

Starkstein, S.E., Migliorelli, R., Teson, A., Petracca, G., Chemerinsky, E., Manes, F., & Leiguarda, R. (1995). Prevalence and clinical correlates of pathological affective display in Alzheimer's disease. *Journal of Neurology Neurosurgery and Psychiatry*, 59, 55–60.

Tortella, F.C., Pellicano, M., & Bowery, N.G. (1989). Dextromethorphan and neuromodulation: old drug coughs up new activities. *TiPS*, 10, 501–507.

Wilson, S.A.K. (1924). Some problems in neurology. II: Pathological laughing and crying. *Journal of Neurology and Psychopathology*, IV, 299–333.

Zeilig, G., Drubach, D.A., Katz-Zeilig, M., & Karatinos, J. (1996). Pathological laughter and crying in patients with closed traumatic brain injury. *Brain Injury*, 10, 591–597.

Zhang, Y., Britto, M.R., Valderhaug, K.L., Wedlund, P.J., & Smith, R.A. (1992). Dextromethorphan: enhancing its systemic availability by way of low-dose quinidine-mediated inhibition of cytochrome P4502D6. *Clinical Pharmacology and Therapeutics*, 51, 647–655.

Progress in Neurotherapeutics and Neuropsychopharmacology, 1:1, 105–113 © 2006 Cambridge University Press
DOI: 10.1017/S1748232105000108   Printed in the United Kingdom

Liquid Fluoxetine versus Placebo for Repetitive Behaviors in Childhood Autism

---

Eric Hollander[1], Erika Swanson[1], Evdokia Anagnostou[1],
Ann Phillips[1], William Chaplin[2] and Stacey Wasserman[1]

[1]*Seaver & New York Autism Center of Excellence, Department of Psychiatry, Mount Sinai School of Medicine, New York, NY*
[2]*Department of Psychology, Saint John's University, Jamaica, New York*

Key words: Autism; liquid fluoxetine; repetitive behaviors; neurotherapeutics; clinical trials; Yale-Brown Obsessive Compulsion Scale.

Introduction and Overview

Autism is a pervasive developmental disorder distinguished by marked deficits in socialization, communication, and repetitive behaviors and/or restricted interests (American Psychiatric Association, 1994). Associated symptoms may include attentional difficulties, impulsivity, aggression, self-injurious behavior, and abnormalities of mood and affect. When broadly defined, approximately 60/10 000 individuals meet criteria for autism, rendering it a considerable concern for families, educators, and health care professionals (Fombonne, 1988). Due to its unknown etiology and heterogeneous presentation in the population, there is no standard pharmacological treatment for autism. However, the core and associated symptoms of autism overlap with other disorders. Therefore, it is possible to develop targeted pharmacological treatments for autism by utilizing medications that effectively treat similar problem behaviors in other disorders (Hollander *et al.*, 2003a).

Repetitive behaviors and restricted interests represent a hallmark symptom domain in autism. However, there appears to be a phenotypic overlap between the repetitive behavior domain in autism and other disorders, such as obsessive–compulsive disorder (OCD). For example, both groups of patients share a rigid adherence to routine and restricted interests. Patients with autism more commonly endorse low-order motoric repetitive behaviors such as tapping, rubbing, ordering,

Correspondence should be addressed to: Eric Hollander, Seaver & NY Autism Center of Excellence, Mount Sinai School of Medicine, Box 1239, One Gustave L. Levy Place, New York, NY 10029; Ph: +212 241 3623; Fax: +212 987 4031; Email: Eric.hollander@mssm.edu.

and hoarding whereas patients with OCD more often report repetitive behaviors such as cleaning, checking, and counting. However, these high-order repetitive behaviors also are endorsed in the autistic population (McDougle *et al.*, 1995). We have reported familial linkage of repetitive behaviors in which autistic children with high levels of repetitive behaviors have higher rates of parents with OCD in comparison to children with low repetitive behaviors (Hollander *et al.*, 2003b). The comorbidity of repetitive behaviors across OCD, autism, and other disorders suggest a common pathophysiology for this symptom domain. We have found striatal abnormalities, specifically increased volume of the right caudate, in 17 adult patients with autism as compared to 17 matched controls. Right caudate and total putamen volumes positively correlated with higher-order repetitive behaviors scores on in the Repetitive and Stereotyped Behaviors domain of the Autism Diagnostic Interview-Revised (ADI-R) (Hollander *et al.*, 2005a). Notably, large volumes of the right caudate have also been reported in adult OCD patients (Scarone *et al.*, 1992).

The repetitive domain in autism may be linked to abnormalities in the 5-hydroxytryptominc (5-HT)/serotonin system. Abrupt reduction of the 5-HT precursor, tryptophan, may increase some repetitive behaviors in autism, such as flapping, pacing, spinning, and self-injury (McDougle *et al.*, 1996a). We found that sensitivity of the 5-HT1d receptor had a specific positive correlation with severity of the repetitive behavior domain but not with severity of other core domains or global functioning (Novotny *et al.*, 2000).

Evidence from positron emission tomography (PET) brain imaging studies also indicates that individuals with autism have abnormal serotonin functions in specific brain regions. In a PET study with radiolabeled 5-HT precursor, alpha C^{11} methyl tryptophan, Chugani *et al.* found decreased 5-HT synthesis in frontal and thalamic regions and increased 5-HT synthesis in contralateral cerebellar dendate regions (Chugani *et al.*, 1997). Consistent with this result was our finding of increased sensitivity of inhibitory 5-HT1d in adult autistic patients as measured by growth hormone (GH) response to sumatriptan, a 5-HT1d receptor agonist (Novotny *et al.*, 2000). Therefore, the mechanism of selective serotonin-reuptake inhibitors (SSRIs) in autism may be an increase in the available synaptic 5-HT via downregulation of inhibitory 5-HT1d autoreceptors.

These findings suggest that repetitive behaviors in autism may be a potential target for SSRI treatment. In the first double-blind, placebo-controlled study of an SSRI in adult autism the results showed that 8 of 15 patients (53%) had significant improvements in repetitive thoughts and behaviors, aggression, social relatedness, and language, compared to none in the placebo group (McDougle *et al.*, 1996b). However, a later trial conducted by the same research team in children and adolescents (mean age: 9.5 years) with autism spectrum disorders (ASD) found poor response to fluvoxamine and notable side-effects in 14 of 18 children on the active medication (McDougle *et al.*, 2000). Only 1 out of the 18 children randomized to fluvoxamine demonstrated clinically significant improvements in the target symptoms. However, it is possible that the reports of early activation symptoms and limited tolerability in these children were related to the high starting dose (50 mg). Open-label trials and case observations suggest that both children and adults may have a better response and greater tolerability when started on low doses of SSRIs, particularly fluoxetine (Fatemi *et al.*, 1998; Markowitz, 1992). A double-blind, placebo-controlled trial of fluoxetine in children and adolescents with autism was needed to validate these preliminary findings.

Trial Rationale

In the current study, we hypothesized that treatment with low-dose liquid fluoxetine would significantly improve the repetitive behaviors domain in children and adolescents with autism.

Clinical Trial

To measure changes in repetitive behaviors, we utilized the compulsion subscale of the Children Yale-Brown Obsessive–Compulsion Scale (CY-BOCS). The CY-BOCS is a variation of the Y-BOCS, adjusted by incorporating basic language for direct administration to young children. In this study ratings were obtained from both the child and caretaker, and only items from the compulsion subscale were assessed. Our secondary hypothesis was that fluoxetine would inadvertently improve global autism severity by reducing the disruption often caused by repetitive behaviors. Global severity was assessed in two ways. First, core autism symptoms, separate from other problem behaviors, were assessed using the Clinical Global Improvement Scale Adapted to Global Autism (CGI-AD). Second, we designed a composite measure that included an assessment of repetitive behaviors as well as the CGI-AD. Repetitive behaviors were measured by calculating a change score for the CY-BOCS (pre-test CY-BOCS–post-test CY-BOCS) and adding this raw score to the CGI-AD measure. Since changes in the communication and socialization domains were thought to be more resistant to treatment with liquid fluoxetine, this composite measure incorporated the hypothesized change in the target behavior, which is more comparable to how the CGI-AD was utilized in other studies (Research Units on Pediatric Psychopharmacology Autism Network, 2002). All CY-BOCS and CGI-AD outcome assessments were completed at baseline and at 4-week intervals by an independent evaluator (IE) who was blind to side-effect data and treatment condition.

    Eligible subjects were between 5 and 17 years of age and met criteria for an ASD. This included subjects who were diagnosed with autism, Asperger Syndrome or

Pervasive Developmental Disorder, Not Otherwise Specified (PDD-NOS). Diagnostic assessments included a structured interview known as the ADI-R, a direct observation assessment called the Autism Diagnostic Observation Schedule-Generic (ADOS-G), and a psychiatric interview to confirm a DSM-IV-TR diagnosis of an ASD. Information about the subject's early language development was collected to make a distinction between Asperger Syndrome and PDD-NOS. Thirty-nine subjects, 30 (76.9%) male and 9 (23.1%) female, ranging in age from 5 to 16 years (mean 8.18 ± 3.04) were included in the analysis (see Table 1).

The study was comprised of three treatment phases: randomized double-blind liquid fluoxetine or placebo treatment for 8 weeks, followed by a 4-week washout period and a subsequent 8-week double-blind, crossover trial. Liquid fluoxetine has an elimination half-life of 2–3 days for the parent and 7–9 days for the metabolite; as such the 4-week washout period between phases (9.3 elimination half-lives for the parent compound, 1.75 elimination half-lives for the metabolite)

Table 1. **Clinical Trial: Patient Characteristics**

CHARACTERISTIC	TOTAL SAMPLE ($n = 39$)	PLACEBO/FLUOXETINE ($n = 20$)	FLUOXETINE/PLACEBO ($n = 19$)
Gender, n (%)			
Male	30 (76.9%)	17 (85%)	13 (68.4%)
Female	9 (23.1%)	3 (15%)	6 (31.6%)
Age (years)			
Mean (±SD)	8.18 (3.0)	7.35 (2.1)	9.1 (3.7)
Range	5–16	5–12	5–16
Ethnicity			
Caucasian	22 (56.4%)	11 (55%)	11 (57.9%)
Asian	2 (5.1%)	1 (5%)	1 (5.3%)
Black	9 (23.1%)	5 (25%)	4 (21.1%)
Hispanic	6 (15.4%)	3 (15%)	3 (15.8%)
Diagnosis			
Autism	34 (87.2%)	17 (85%)	71 (89.5%)
As pergers	5 (12.8%)	3 (15%)	2 (10.5%)
Clinical global impressions scale (by independent evaluator)			
Autism severity (±SD)	4.6 (0.9%)	4.5 (0.84)	4.7 (0.9)
C-YBOCS (by independent evaluator)			
Mean (±SD)	13.2 (2.7)	13.5 (2.9)	12.8 (2.6)
Range	8–18	8–18	8–16
IQ[a]			
Mean (±SD)	63.7 (27.9)	68.1 (26.7)	59.2 (29.1)
Range	30–132	30–111	33–132
Vineland adaptive behavior composite[a]			
Mean (±SD)	46.6 (21.9)	47.9 (19.4)	45.1 (24.6)
Range	20–110	20–107	20–110

$p < 0.07$ for all comparisons.
[a] Total sample $n = 34$, $n = 17$ for both conditions.
Source: Hollander *et al.* (2005b).

was not long enough to guarantee complete elimination of the metabolite. However, we attempted to balance the burden on the patient with the complete elimination of the metabolite.

The dosing schedule began at 2.5 mg/day of liquid fluoxetine or placebo once a day for 1 week. The following 7 weeks followed a flexible titration schedule based on weight, tolerability, and side-effects up to a maximum dose of 0.8 mg/kg/day (0.3 mg/kg for week 2, 0.5 mg/kg/day for week 3, and 0.8 mg/kg/day for weeks 4–8). The dose prescribed on day 28 (end of week 4) was sustained until the end of the 8-week phase, unless reduction was clinically indicated due to reported side-effects. The mean maximum dose for fluoxetine over the course of the study was 10.6 ± 3.65 mg (range 4.8–20 mg) or 0.38 ± 0.97 mg/kg versus 11.1 ± 4.47 mg fluoxetine equivalents (range 4.8–30 mg), or 0.4 ± 0.11 mg/kg for the placebo. The mean final dose for fluoxetine was 9.9 mg $+ 4.35$ (range 2.4–20 mg), or 0.36 ± 0.116 mg/kg versus 10.8 ± 4.7 mg equivalents (range 4.8–30 mg), or 0.36 ± 0.15 mg/kg for the placebo. There was a significant correlation between age and dose, with older children getting higher doses ($r = 0.72$, $p < 0.001$ for placebo, and $r = 0.58$, $p < 0.001$ for fluoxetine).

It was also important to investigate the tolerability of fluoxetine versus placebo in this young population. At each visit, the treating clinician inquired about side-effects using the Fluoxetine Side-Effects Checklist (FSEC). This checklist systematically reviewed each major biological system through a series of 63 items. Due to concerns about suicidality and agitation, the Suicidality subscale of the Overt Aggression Scale-Modified (OAS-M) was also completed at each visit. The analysis revealed that side-effects did not significantly or marginally differ between liquid fluoxetine and placebo (Table 1). It is important to note that there was no trend or significant effect of drug versus placebo on the suicide subscale of the OAS-M.

Conclusions

The results of this study suggest that liquid fluoxetine was superior to placebo in reducing repetitive behaviors in autism as measured by the CY-BOCS. There was a significant drug by time effect, with a medium to large effect size (0.76). A significant linear trend $\times$ treatment interaction was obtained ($z = -2.075$, $se = 0.407$, $p = 0.038$). There were general linear and quadratic trends in the data in both the placebo and fluoxetine conditions but the linear decrease was significantly greater in the fluoxetine than in the placebo condition. These results are shown graphically in Figure 1 in which the values of the actual means and standard errors on the CY-BOCS are presented. Table 2 describes the means and standard deviations for both drug condition and phase order.

The effect of fluoxetine on reducing global measures of ASD was not significant, however this may be due to the statistical emphasis of the composite measure on

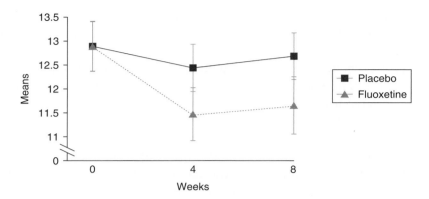

Fig. 1.
Effect of fluoxetine/placebo on repetitive behaviors (CY-BOCS compulsion score). Source: Hollander *et al.* (2005b).

Table 2. **Means for Primary Outcome Measures**

		CONDITION 1						CONDITION 2					
		Phase I --- Phase II						Phase I --- Phase II					
		Placebo			*Fluoxetine*			*Fluoxetine*			**Placebo**		
	Week	0	4	8	12	16	20	0	4	8	12	16	20
CY-BOCS	Mean	13.45	12.7	12.95	12.93	11.94	11.77	12.84	11.05	11.63	12.24	12.13	12.38
	SD	2.9	3.2	3.2	3.5	3.4	3.2	2.6	3.4	3.8	3.5	2.6	2.4
CGI-AD improvement	Mean			3.58			3.06			3.42			3.19
	SD			0.8			1.1			1.2			1
Global composite improvement	Mean			3.21			1.73			2.21			3.50
	SD			2.6			3.6			3.0			3.0

Source: Hollander *et al.* (2005b).

the social and communication domains, which were less likely to show improvement over the 8-week period. Also, the crossover study design introduced a phase order effect may have biased the CGI-AD since subjects in both groups showed more improvement in the second phase. This phase order effect may have been partly due to the fact that the 4-week washout phase allowed only for 1.75 half-lives of the metabolite. Still, our global composite measure did approach statistical significance for fluoxetine ($p = 0.056$) and 19 of our 34 subjects (56%) showed a global composite improvement score of 2 (much improved) or better on fluoxetine. Given these results, we can postulate that the effect of fluoxetine on global autism severity may be clinically meaningful. Earlier studies in autistic adults treated with fluvoxamine and clomipramine with a parallel design and similar sample size had stronger findings (McDougle *et al.*, 1996b; Gordon *et al.*, 1993). However this may have been attributed to greater tolerability of adults to high doses of SSRIs or a greater severity of repetitive behaviors at baseline.

Influence on the Field

This study had several limitations. First, the brevity of the trial restricts our understanding to the short-term effect of liquid fluoxetine in autism. Long maintenance trials will be needed to evaluate long-term trajectories and side-effects of fluoxetine treatment. Second, while the crossover design of the study allowed for within-subject comparison it also caused phase order effects, which may have partially masked differences on the global autism measure. Also, due to the low doses of fluoxetine used in this study these results may not accurately represent the effects of individuals on higher doses. Lastly, since our population was confined to rather high functioning children and adolescents who were 5 years and older, future trials should stratify for lower-functioning autism populations and younger children, since SSRIs may encourage neurogenesis (Gaspar *et al.*, 2003) and differentiation in early brain development, or may imitate the serotonin peak in the brain observed in typically developing toddlers and missing in young children with autism (Chugani *et al.*, 1999). Lastly, future studies should systematically assess improvements in the other core symptoms domains (e.g. communication and socialization) as well as associated problem behaviors.

This study was the first double-blind, placebo-controlled crossover study of the effects of liquid fluoxetine in children and adolescents with autism. The findings provide support for the efficacy of fluoxetine in the treatment of repetitive behaviors, and perhaps global symptoms, in children and adolescents with autism. In contrast to side-effects associated with clomipramine in children with autism such as sedation, weight gain, cardiac complications, and lowering of the seizure threshold, we found no differences in side-effects in fluoxetine versus placebo. Given concerns about increased suicidality in children treated with SSRIs, it is important to note that we found no increase in the suicide subscale of the OAS-M, and in fact, patients on fluoxetine reported less anxiety/nervousness than placebo.

Despite study limitations, the data suggests that fluoxetine may be an effective and well-tolerated medication for the treatment of children and adolescents with autism. To date, no medications have been shown to reduce overall autistic symptoms. Therefore, the current pharmacological approach is to utilize medications that target specific core and associated symptoms and to evaluate the risk-benefit ratio of these treatments for each individual patient. The findings of this study are an important contribution to the literature as they provide support for the use of fluoxetine as a targeted treatment for the repetitive behavior domain of autism and verify the safety of this drug in young populations.

References

American Psychiatric Association. (1994). *Diagnostic and Statistical Manual of Mental Disorders* (4th ed.). Washington, DC: American Psychiatric Association.

Chugani, D.C., Muzik, O., Rothermel, R., Behen, M., Chakraborty, P., Mangner, T., da Silva, E.A., & Chugani, H.T. (1997). Altered serotonin synthesis in the dentathalmocortical pathway in autistic boys. *Annals of Neurology*, 42, 666–669.

Chugani, D.C., Muzik, O., Behen, M., Rothermel, R., Janisse, J.J., Lee, J., & Chugani, H.T. (1999). Developmental changes in brain serotonin synthesis capacity in autistic and nonautistic children. *Annals of Neurology*, 45, 287–295.

Fatemi, S.H., Realmuto, G.M., Khan, L., & Thuras, P. (1998). Fluoxetine in treatment of adolescent patients with autism: a longitudinal open trial. *Journal of Autism and Developmental Disorders*, 28, 303–307.

Fombonne, E. (1988). Epidemiology of the pervasive developmental disorders. *Trends in Evidence-Based Neuropsychiatry*, 5, 29–36.

Gaspar, P., Cases, O., & Maroteaux, L. (2003). The developmental role of serotonin: news from mouse molecular genetics. *Nature Reviews Neuroscience*, 4, 1002–1012.

Gordon, C.T., State, R.C., Nelson, J.E., Hamburger, S.D., & Rapoport, J.L. (1993). A double-blind comparison of clomiprimine, despramine, and placebo in the treatment of autistic disorder. *Archives of General Psychiatry*, 50, 441–447.

Hollander, E., Phillips, A.T., & Yeh, C. (2003a). Targeted treatments for symptom domains in child and adolescent autism. *Lancet*, 362, 222–252.

Hollander, E., King, A., Delaney, K., Smith, C.J., & Silverman, J.M. (2003b). Obsessive–compulsive behaviors in parents of multiplex autism families. *Psychiatry Research*, 117, 11–16.

Hollander, E., Anagnostou, E., Chaplin, W., Esposito, K., Haznedar, M.M., Licalzi, E., Wasserman, S., Soorya, L., & Buchsbaum, M. (2005a). Striatal volume on magnetic resonance imaging and repetitive behaviors in autism. *Biological Psychiatry*, 58, 226–232.

Hollander, E., Phillips, A., Chaplin, W., Zagursky, K., Novotny, S., Wasserman, S., & Iyengar, R. (2005b). A placebo-controlled crossover trial of liquid fluoxetine on repetitive behaviors in childhood and adolescent autism. *Neuropsychopharmacology*, 30, 582–589. Reprinted with permission.

Markowitz, P.I. (1992). Effect of fluoxetine on self-injurious behavior in the developmentally disabled: a preliminary study. *Journal of Clinical Psychopharmacology*, 12, 27–31.

McDougle, C.J., Kresch, L.E., Goodman, W.K., Naylor, S.T., Volkmar, F.R., Cohen, D.J., & Price, L.H. (1995). A case controlled study of repetitive thoughts and behavior in adults with autistic disorder and obsessive–compulsive disorder. *American Journal of Psychiatry*, 152, 772–777.

McDougle, C.J., Naylor, S.T., Cohen, D.J., Aghajanian, G.K., Heninger, G.R., & Price, L.H. (1996a). Effects of tryptophan depletion in drug-free adults with autistic disorder. *Archives of General Psychiatry*, 53, 993–1000.

McDougle, C.J., Naylor, S.T., Cohen, D.J., Volkmar, F.R., Heninger, G.R., & Price, L.H. (1996b). A double-blind, placebo-controlled study of fluvoxamine in adults with autistic disorder. *Archives of General Psychiatry*, 53, 1001–1008.

McDougle, C.J., Kresch, L.E., & Posey, D.J. (2000). Repetitive thoughts and behavior in pervasive developmental disorders: treatment with serotonin reuptake inhibitors. *Journal of Autism and Developmental Disorders*, 30, 427–435.

Novotny, S., Hollander, E., Allen, A., Mosovich, S., Aronowitz, B., Cartwright, C., DeCaria, C., & Dolgoff-Kaspar, R. (2000). Increased growth hormone response to sumatriptan challenge in adult autistic disorders. *Psychiatry Research*, 94, 173–177.

Research Units on Pediatric Psychopharmacology Autism Network. (2002). Risperidone in children with autism and serious behavioral problems. *New England Journal of Medicine*, 347, 314–321.

Scarone, S., Colombo, C., Livian, S., Abbruzzese, M., Ronchi, P., Locatelli, M., Scotti, G., & Smeraldi, E. (1992). Increased right caudate nucleus size in obsessive–compulsive disorder: detection with magnetic resonance imaging. *Psychiatry Research*, 45, 115–121.

Progress in Neurotherapeutics and Neuropsychopharmacology, 1:1, 115–120 © 2006 Cambridge University Press
DOI: 10.1017/S174823210500011X   Printed in the United Kingdom

Testing Multiple Novel Mechanisms for Treating Schizophrenia in a Single Trial

---

Herbert Y. Meltzer

Department of Psychiatry, Vanderbilt University School of Medicine, Nashville, TN, USA;
Email: herbert.meltzer@vanderbilt.edu

Key words: Schizophrenia; clinical trial; osanetrant; NK3 antagonist; 5-HT2A/C antagonist; central cannabinoid antagonist; neurotensin antagonist.

Introduction

Schizophrenia is one of the most common and severe forms of mental illness. Its major features include psychosis, cognitive impairment, negative symptoms, and a high rate of suicide, the latter mainly due to depression and hopelessness. The treatment of schizophrenia in much of the world is largely pharmacologic, with psychosocial support and cognitive rehabilitation quite useful, but often not provided because of cost. Prior to the reintroduction of clozapine in 1990 in the USA, the major pharmacologic treatment for schizophrenia was dopamine D_2 receptor blockers, such as haloperidol, whose chief side-effects were mechanism-based blockade of D_2 receptors in the dorsal striatum, leading to a variety of acute and chronic extrapyramidal side-effects (EPS) (e.g. tardive dyskinesia). The demonstration that clozapine was more efficacious in a subgroup of patients and produced fewer EPS of all types (Meltzer, 1997; Kane *et al.*, 1988), led to search for other drugs which were clozapine like but did not produce agranulocytosis, the side-effect which limited clozapine to use in treatment-resistant patients. The ensuing decade produced a variety of clozapine-like drugs, based on the principle of some dopamine D_2 receptor blockade, accompanied by serotonin (5-HT)$_{2A}$ or 5-HT$_{1A}$, partial agonism, or both (Meltzer, 2001). The introduction of olanzapine, quetiapine, risperidone, ziprasidone, and zotepine has led to their replacing the D_2 blockers as first-line therapy. Recently, a partial dopamine D_2/D_3 agonist mechanism accompanied by 5-HT$_{1A}$ partial agonism, and 5-HT$_{2A}$ antagonism (i.e. aripiprazole) has

Correspondence should be addressed to: Herbert Y. Meltzer, MD, Department of Psychiatry, Vanderbilt University School of Medicine, Psychiatric Hospital at Vanderbilt, 1601 23rd Ave South Nashville, TN 37212, USA, Ph: +615 327 7049; Email: herbert.meltzer@vanderbilt.edu.

been found to have similar advantages to drugs like risperidone. Despite the advantages of these drugs, particularly for cognition (Woodward *et al.*, 2005) and low EPS, they are far from fully effective for the majority of patients with schizophrenia and some members of the class, especially olanzapine and clozapine, produce serious metabolic side-effects (Meltzer, 2005).

For these reasons, there is an intensive search for novel mechanism to treat schizophrenia, particularly drugs which can address those domains of the illness which are least improved by the available agents; for example, cognitive impairment and negative symptoms, or positive symptoms in those patients who fail to respond to other antipsychotic drugs, including clozapine. Basic research concerning the nature of the biologic deficit in schizophrenia, the mechanism of action of available agents for schizophrenia or cognitive impairment, the biological basis of cognition and motivation, and genetic studies, to name the most important, have provided a broad array of targets for novel treatment (Roth & Xia, 2004). Preclinical *in vitro* and *in vivo* studies can provide useful screens for promising mechanisms, ultimately leading to best candidates for human studies. Following safety studies (Phase I), clinical studies in patients are needed to obtain proof of concept. While all phases of this process are costly, the most costly is the last stage (Phase III), with the average cost per patient for an initial 4–6 weeks study in patients averaging $25 000 to $35 000 per patient. The typical design involves one–two doses of the test compound, an active comparator, and a placebo. The latter is necessary to show that the trial is valid by demonstrating greater efficacy in the active comparator or the test compound. With 60–90 patients per group, such studies can easily cost $8 to $12 000 000.

Novel Trial Design

This is the background for the special interest in a recently published study, which examined the antipsychotic efficacy and safety for the treatment of schizophrenia, of four novel compounds versus haloperidol, the active comparator, and placebo (Meltzer *et al.*, 2004). None of the four compounds had ever previously been studied in schizophrenia. Due to the multiple drug comparisons, it has been referred to as a "metatrial". This design reduced the number of subjects needed to be exposed to placebo, facilitated a comparison of the four compounds with one another, although that was not its primary goal, and reduced the cost of studying any one drug by 33%, by utilizing common placebo and comparator groups. Since only a single dose of each drug was studied, with limited information to justify that dose, conclusions about efficacy, let alone relative efficacy, were necessarily tentative. The four investigational drugs studied were osanetant, a NK_3 antagonist (SR142801), a 5-HT2$_{A/C}$ antagonist (SR46349B), a central cannabinoid (CB_1) antagonist (SR141716), and a neurotensin (NTS_1) antagonist (SR48692). The doses of the investigational drugs were chosen based on tolerability data, or in the case of the 5-HT2$_{A/C}$ antagonist, a positron emission tomography (PET) study. The rationale for studying these compounds is given elsewhere (Meltzer *et al.*, 2004). Preclinical studies suggest that NK$_3$ antagonists provide a novel way to reduce limbic dopaminergic activity (Spooren *et al.*, in press). The 5-HT$_{2A/2C}$ antagonist was known to mimic a key aspect of the pharmacology of clozapine, without any D$_2$ receptor blockade (Bonaccorso *et al.*, 2002) while the CB$_1$ antagonist was of interest because of its ability to block amphetamine-induced locomotor activity (Poncelet *et al.*, 1999). The choice of a neurotensin antagonist to treat schizophrenia was controversial because the majority of evidence suggests that a neurotensin agonist might be more likely to be clinically effective than an antagonist (Boules *et al.*, 2005).

Methods

In the metatrial, patients with a diagnosis of schizophrenia or schizoaffective disorder were required to be hospitalized at baseline and through day 15 after randomization. Eligible patients were also required to have a total Positive and Negative Scale for Schizophrenia (PANSS; Kay *et al.*, 1987) score greater than 65 (moderate severity) at screening and baseline, including a minimum score of 4 (moderate), on at least two of four PANSS positive symptom items (delusions, conceptual disorganization, hallucinatory behavior, and suspiciousness). The study was completed in 50 US centers, divided into six groups, with 7–11 centers per group: two protocols, that is, two of the novel drugs, placebo, and haloperidol arms, were allocated to each group of centers. Following screening, and a 2- to 10-day single-blind placebo lead-in period, 481 eligible patients were randomized to receive once daily treatment with one of the investigational drugs, haloperidol (10 mg/day), or placebo for 6 weeks in a 3 : 1 : 1 ratio. The final numbers were placebo or haloperidol ($N = 98$ per group) and 69–74 for each of the four experimental drug groups. The duration of the trial was 6 weeks.

Results

The percentages of patients completing the study was highest for the NK$_3$ antagonist (43%) group and lowest in the placebo (20%) and CB$_1$ antagonist (21%) groups, with completion rates for the other three groups ranging from 31% to 35%. While this is a low completion rate for a study of this kind, it was sufficient to provide analyzable data, using a last observation carried forward analysis. The most common reason for withdrawal was lack of efficacy, and the highest rates of withdrawal for this reason were in the CB$_1$ antagonist, NTS$_1$ antagonist, and placebo groups. Few patients withdrew due to adverse events, and these withdrawal rates were similar across the treatment groups.

The haloperidol-treated group, compared to placebo treatment, showed significantly greater improvements at 6 weeks in four primary efficacy measures: (1) the total PANSS score; (2) the derived total score for the Brief Psychiatric Rating Scale (BPRS); (3) its positive symptom subscale (consisting of delusions, hallucinations, conceptual disorganization, and bizarre behavior); and (4) the Clinical Global Impression Scale. The magnitude of the improvement in total PANSS score in the haloperidol-treated group at 6 weeks was $14.0 \pm SD19.9$, similar to that of other clinical trials of schizophrenia, supporting the validity of the study. The other drugs with greater than placebo effects on the PANSS total were the $5\text{-HT}_{2A/2C}$ antagonist, SR43469B (-10.2 ± 18.4), and the NK_3 antagonist, osanetant (-9.8 ± 17.5). The improvement in the haloperidol-treated patients was not significantly different from that with osanetant or SR43469B. There were no statistically significant differences between the NK_3 antagonist group and the placebo group for positive or negative symptoms. However, there was a relationship between median plasma concentration and decrease from baseline in BPRS total score, suggesting that higher dosage, producing higher plasma levels, might be more efficacious, assuming no problem with tolerability.

In the $5\text{-HT}_{2A/2C}$ antagonist group, mean reductions in the PANSS negative subscale, PANSS general psychopathology subscale, Calgary Depression Scale, and Clinical Global Impression of Improvement (CGI-I) scores were significantly greater than those in the placebo group. However, these reductions were smaller than those seen in the haloperidol group. There was no association between median plasma concentration and decrease from baseline in BPRS total scores for SR43469B.

There were no statistically significant differences between either the CB_1 antagonist group or the NTS_1 antagonist group, and the placebo group for any of the efficacy variables. The negative data with the latter two compounds provides further support for the validity of the study but does not rule out that these compounds might have some benefit at different doses or in a different population of patients with schizophrenia.

EPS, including akathisia and abnormal involuntary movements, occurred at a significantly higher rate in the haloperidol-treated group than in the placebo-treated group but not in any of the four novel drug groups. Headache, insomnia, psychosis, and agitation were the most frequently occurring adverse events. Weight gain was not notable in any of the drug treatment groups.

Discussion

The major results of this trial were that the novel concept of a "metatrial" to simultaneously compare efficacy and tolerability of multiple, novel antipsychotic compounds was validated and that two of the compounds, an NK_3 antagonist

(SR142801) and a 5-HT$_{2A/2C}$ antagonist (SR46349B), had sufficient efficacy and tolerability, albeit in somewhat different domains, to warrant further study. The study provided sufficient information for power analyses for future studies with these drugs and for further exploration of clinically effective doses. Only further clinical studies with these compounds and the two which failed will validate the conclusions of this study. On the basis of this study, a second trial was initiated with osanetant. The details of dosage, design, etc. are not available at this time. However, in this trial, osanetant failed to be as effective as risperidone (Arvanitis, 9/01/2005, personal communication), but it is not yet known if it again differentiated from placebo. It could be that the pharmacokinetic features of this compound are not ideal. Another NK$_3$ antagonist, talnetant, is being extensively studied for schizophrenia. There is preliminary indication that it is effective to improve positive symptoms and cognition, and that these are dose related (Lowy, 6/01/2005, personal communication). There is, to my knowledge, no further research in schizophrenia with SR43469B, but a similar compound, ACP-103, is being studied for this indication. This compound has proven useful, as monotherapy, to treat L-Dopa psychosis (Davis, 6/15/2005, personal communication).

Conclusion

In summary, the concept of testing multiple putative antipsychotic agents for the schizophrenia indication in a single trial was given its initial test in this study. From multiple perspectives, the design appears to have been adequate to improve clinically useful information.

Acknowledgement

Supported, in part, by a grant from the William K. Warren Medical Research Foundation and the Ritter Foundation.

References

Bonaccorso, S., Meltzer, H.Y., Li, Z., Dai, J., Alboszta, A.R., & Ichikawa, J. (2002). SR46349-B, a 5HT$_2$ receptor antagonist, potentiates haloperidol-induced dopamine release in rat medial prefrontal cortex via 5HT$_{1A}$ receptor activation. *Neuropsychopharmacology*, 27, 430–441.

Boules, M., Fredrickson, P., & Richelson, E. (2005). Neurotensin agonists as an alternative to antipsychotics. *Expert Opinion Investigational Drugs*, 4, 359–369.

Kane, J., Honigfeld, G., Singer, J., & Meltzer, H.Y. (1988). The Clozaril Collaborative Study Group. Clozapine for the treatment-resistant schizophrenic: a double-blind comparison with chlorpromazine. *Archives of General Psychiatry*, 45, 789–796.

Kay, S.R., Fiszbein, A., & Opler, L.A. (1987). The Positive and Negative Syndrome Scale (PANSS) for schizophrenia. *Schizophrenia Bull*, 13, 261–276.

Meltzer, H.Y. (1997). Treatment-resistant schizophrenia – the role of clozapine. *Current Medical Research and Opinion*, 14(1), 1–20.

Meltzer, H.Y. (2001). Serotonin as a target for antipsychotic drug action. In: Breier, A., Tran, P., Herrea, J.M., Tollefson, G.D., & Bymaster, F.P. (eds.), *Current Issues in the Psychopharmacology of Schizophrenia*, Chapter 17. Philadelphia: Lippincott Williams & Wilkins Healthcare, pp. 289–303.

Meltzer, H.Y. (2005). The metabolic consequences of long-term treatment with olanzapine, quetiapine and risperidone: are there differences? *International Journal of Neuropsychopharmacology*, 8, 153–156.

Meltzer, H.Y., Arvanitis, L., Bauer, D., & Rein, W. (2004). A placebo-controlled evaluation of four novel compounds for the treatment of schizophrenia and schizoaffective disorder. *American Journal of Psychiatry*, 161, 975–984.

Poncelet, M., Barnouin, M.C., Breliere, J.C., Le Fur, G., & Soubrie, P. (1999). Blockade of cannabinoid (CB1) receptors by 141716 selectively antagonizes drug-induced reinstatement of exploratory behaviour in gerbils. *Psychopharmacology (Berl)*, 144 (2),144–150.

Roth, B.L., & Xia, Z. (2004). Molecular and cellular mechanisms for the polarized sorting of serotonin receptors: relevance for genesis and treatment of psychosis. *Critical Reviews in Neurobiology*, 16, 229–236.

Spooren, W., Riemer, C., & Meltzer, H.Y. (in press). NK$_3$ receptor antagonists: the next generation of anti-psychotics? *Nature Reviews Drug Discovery*, 2005; 4: 967–975

Woodward, N.D., Purdon, S.E., Meltzer, H.Y., & Zald, D.H. (2005). A meta-analysis of neuropsychological change to clozapine, olanzapine, quetiapine, and risperidone in schizophrenia. *International Journal of Neuropsychopharmacolgy*, 8, 1–16.

Progress in Neurotherapeutics and Neuropsychopharmacology, 1:1, 121–131 © 2006 Cambridge University Press
DOI: 10.1017/S1748232105000121   Printed in the United Kingdom

Selegiline in the Treatment of Negative Symptoms of Schizophrenia

Allison Lin and J. Alexander Bodkin

Clinical Psychopharmacology Research Program, McLean Hospital, Harvard Medical School;
Email: abodkin@mclean.harvard.edu

Key words: Selegiline; schizophrenia; negative symptoms; neurotherapeutics; clinical trial.

Introduction and Overview

One of the great successes of modern psychiatry was the introduction of antipsychotic drugs over 50 years ago (Ayd & Blackwell, 1970). The impressive effectiveness of these agents in relieving florid positive symptoms of schizophrenia has permitted a whole population of formerly institutionalized patients to live in the community. Unfortunately, this great benefit has not been matched by the effect of antipsychotic drugs on the negative symptoms of schizophrenia, which so limit the daily function of these patients, and classical neuroleptics often worsened these symptoms. More recently, atypical antipsychotics have shown improved properties in this regard, but negative symptoms remain the least medication-responsive features of chronic schizophrenia.

The impoverishment of emotion and initiative that underlie negative symptoms resemble symptoms affecting patients with Parkinson's disease, as well as the pseudo-parkinsonian effects of first-generation antipsychotics, and has been hypothesized to reflect specific deficits in the functioning of dopaminergic pathways (Bermanzohn & Siris, 1992; Davis *et al.*, 1991). Selegiline (formerly l-deprenyl) is a dopamine enhancing antiparkinsonian drug (Knoll, 1983), which acts as a selective monoamine oxidase type B (MAO-B) inhibitor without the clinical toxicities that have limited the use of non-selective MAO inhibitors (MAOIs) in psychiatry. The potential of selegiline to alleviate some of the parkinsonian-like emotional deficits of schizophrenics has led to a series of investigations of its use as a specific remedy for negative symptoms over the past 15 years. This article presents the results of the

Correspondence should be addressed to: J. Alexander Bodkin, MD, McLean Hospital, 115 Mill Street, Belmont, MA 02478, 617 855 2000; Email: abodkin@mclean.harvard.edu

largest and most extended trial yet carried out, using a multi-center, double-blind, placebo-controlled, parallel group design over 12 weeks to test the efficacy of selegiline in treating the negative symptoms of schizophrenic outpatients stabilized on chronic antipsychotic medication (Bodkin *et al.*, 2005). The results support the hypothesis that selegiline is effective in moderating negative symptoms without introducing the burden of adverse effects associated with non-selective MAOIs, and without heightening positive symptoms.

Schizophrenic symptomatology is often characterized as having separate positive and negative dimensions. Positive symptoms include delusions and hallucination, and represent the more conspicuous and socially disruptive features of the illness. Negative symptoms denote a cluster of deficits in schizophrenic patients, encompassing affective flattening, apathy, anergia, anhedonia, cognitive impairment and poverty of speech (Carpenter *et al.*, 1988; Andreasen, 1982).

The clinical overlap between the domain of negative symptoms, extrapyramidal, and depressive symptoms has been noted for many years. Akinesia has been proposed as the shared central features of Parkinson's disease, retarded depression, and negative symptoms of schizophrenia, with dopaminergic hypofunction as its underlying mechanism (Bermanzohn & Siris, 1992). This has specific therapeutic implications, and avoids the complexities of subtyping specific etiologies of patients presenting with these symptoms, that is, intrinsic neural deficits (Carpenter *et al.*, 1988); versus pseudoparkinsonism (Rifkin *et al.*, 1975); versus depression (Siris *et al.*, 1978).

Current treatments for negative symptoms center on the atypical antipsychotics, with clozapine serving as the benchmark and prototype (Kane *et al.*, 1988). In comparison to traditional antipsychotics, the atypicals are much less likely to cause extrapyramidal symptoms, but with the exception of clozapine, may be somewhat less effective than classical neuroleptics in controlling psychotic symptoms – leading to their widespread use in combination with each other – and they are associated with problematic metabolic side-effects not found with classical neuroleptics (Wirshing, 2001).

In addition to the atypical antipsychotics, antidepressants have been explored as adjunctive treatments in schizophrenia for many years (Siris *et al.*, 1978) and there have been several studies of selective serotonin reuptake inhibitors (SSRI) antidepressants with promising results (e.g. Goff *et al.*, 1995; Silver & Nassar, 1992). However, this approach has not become widely established, and may be effective only in a subgroup of schizophrenics with concurrent depressive symptoms. A similar subgroup-specific effect has been suggested in patients with symptoms of anxiety, who respond to benzodiazepines (Bodkin, 1990; Adan & Siris, 1989).

The hypothesis that regional dopamine hypofunction may underlie the cluster of negative symptoms in schizophrenia suggests the possible benefit of the use of a dopamine agonist in conjunction with the antipsychotic regimen (Davis *et al.*,

1991; Levi-Minzi *et al.*, 1991). The minimal adverse effects of selegiline and its mood-buoying effects encourage its use in this role (Bodkin, 1990).

The effectiveness of MAOIs particularly in patients with atypical depression and anxiety has long been recognized (Klein *et al.*, 1980). Though MAOIs are associated with the treatment of primary mood and anxiety disorders exclusively, they were first studied not in depression or anxiety, but on institutionalized schizophrenics, in whom a mild beneficial activating effect was noted (Kamman *et al.*, 1953). However, it was subsequently observed that these drugs would often exacerbate psychotic symptoms (Cole *et al.*, 1961). Although, several subsequent studies have demonstrated improvements in negative symptoms without over stimulation when the non-selective MAOI tranylcypromine was combined with antipsychotic medications (Bucci, 1987), the great care that must be taken in using MAOIs in this population has completely discouraged their use.

Purpose of Trial

We sought to test the efficacy of selegiline at an MAO-B selective dosage, in treating the negative symptoms of schizophrenia. Several open label trials have been promising (Gupta *et al.*, 1999; Bodkin *et al.*, 1996; Perenyi *et al.*, 1991), but two small, brief placebo-controlled trials yielded negative results (Jungerman *et al.*, 1999; Goff *et al.*, 1993). We sought to conduct a better-powered placebo-controlled trial using a more adequate duration of treatment, to more conclusively test the drug's effectiveness for this often clinically intractable condition.

Agent

Selegiline was synthesized in the 1960s by a Hungarian group headed by Joseph Knoll in an effort to develop an MAOI that would provide the antidepressant activity of available agents, without the risk of hypertensive crisis from the consumption of foods high in tyramine (Knoll, 1983). The levorotatory isomer was found to be a selective MAO-B inhibitor at doses below 20 mg/day, and thus free of any tyramine interaction, but unfortunately at these doses it was not reliably effective as an antidepressant (Bodkin & Kwon, 2001). Subsequently, it was shown to be an effective antidepressant at non-selective oral doses (30–60 mg/day) (Bodkin & Kwon, 2001) including in the subset of patients with treatment-refractory depression (Mann *et al.*, 1989). Most remarkably, the side-effect profile of selegiline given at extremely high doses even to elderly depressed patients has been shown to differ little from placebo (Bodkin & Kwon, 2001). Currently, selegiline is FDA approved only for the adjunctive treatment of L-dopa-refractory Parkinson's disease. In addition to alleviating motor symptoms, the drug has been observed to have mood elevating and bradyphrenia-alleviating effects in parkinsonian patients (Lees, 1991). It has been suggested that selegiline treatment slows the progression of Parkinson's disease (Tetrud & Langston, 1989), although this has been controversial (Mandel *et al.*, 2003). More recently, the transdermal administration of selegiline has been tested in the treatment of depression and found effective (Bodkin & Amsterdam, 2002) at doses not increasing tyramine sensitivity (Amsterdam, 2003).

Several open trials with low-dose selegiline have suggested benefit for schizophrenic patients with negative symptoms. The first trial was conducted with 13 male chronic schizophrenic patients who were given selegiline to on-going neuroleptic treatment (Perenyi *et al.*, 1992). A significant improvement was found on the Negative Symptom Rating Scale and on the anergia factor of the Brief Psychiatric Rating Scale (BPRS). A second study was published in 1996, with 21 patients meeting criteria for schizophrenia or schizoaffective disorder who displayed prominent negative symptoms (Bodkin *et al.*, 1996). After 6 weeks adjunctive treatment with selegiline, patients exhibited reductions in depressive and extrapyramidal symptoms accompanying a 34.7% reduction in negative symptoms as measured on the Scale for the Assessment of Negative Symptoms (SANS). Importantly, selegiline treatment was not associated with increased severity of positive symptoms. Subsequently Gupta and colleagues published a case series including three patients in continuing day treatment, who each received low-dose selegiline augmentation of on-going antipsychotic treatment (Gupta *et al.*, 1999). All three patients demonstrated improvement in negative symptoms, particularly through a "broader range of affect" and increased motivation.

Two small placebo-controlled studies have indicated no benefit of selegiline over inactive control in treating negative symptoms. Jungerman and colleagues studied 16 schizophrenic patients given 15 mg daily over 8 weeks in addition to continued neuroleptic treatment (Jungerman *et al.*, 1999). The study reported no specific drug effect, but a large placebo effect. This was hypothesized to be due to the increased doctor–patient contact during the study. Another group studied 33 schizophrenic patients, half of them treated with selegiline adjunctively for 6 weeks for tardive dyskinesia, half with matched placebo (Goff *et al.*, 1993). Negative symptoms were rated pre- and post-treatment, as a secondary measure. It was reported that patients receiving selegiline displayed less improvement of tardive dyskinesia than to those receiving placebo and no difference was found between groups in improvement of negative symptoms.

Clinical Trial

We recruited 67 clinically stable schizophrenic outpatients at three sites (McLean Hospital in Belmont, MA; Hillside Hospital in Glen Oaks, NY; and Creedmoor Hospital in Queens, NY) who demonstrated prominent negative symptoms, and no more than moderate positive symptoms. Subjects were randomized to placebo or

5 mg bid selegiline. Participants were required to remain on fixed doses of all psychotropic medication, with the exception of pro re nata (prn) benzodiazepines, which were permitted at clinician discretion. Inclusion criteria included a total SANS score $\geqslant 12$, with at least two global subscale scores $\geqslant 3$; antipsychotic treatment $\geqslant 1$ year, at the current dose $\geqslant 1$ month, with any other psychotropic medications at a constant dose $\geqslant 1$ month. Exclusion criteria included a score $\geqslant 5$ on any BPRS thinking disturbance item; treatment within 1 month of screening with antidepressant medication; or a current diagnosis of major mood or substance abuse disorder.

After screening, subjects were evaluated every 2 weeks for 3 months using the SANS, BPRS, Hamilton Depression Rating Scale (HDRS), Simpson–Angus Rating Scale, and Clinical Global Impressions of severity (CGI-S) and of change (CGI-I). The patient sample was characterized by relatively long and severe courses of illness and relatively high dosages of neuroleptics. Random effects regression models were used for analysis with repeated measures taken within subjects while controlling for baseline levels of each clinical measure and visit sequence. Statistical significance required two-tailed $p < 0.05$.

Results

Among 67 patients receiving at least one dose of active medication, changes favoring selegiline over placebo were found on SANS summary total, avolition-apathy and anhedonia global scores; BPRS total; and CGI-S and CGI-I. There was no worsening of positive symptoms, as measured by the BPRS thought disturbance factor. No difference emerged between groups in changes on the Simpson–Angus Ratings EPS scale or BPRS thinking disturbance factor. Treatment effects did not differ by site or gender in random effects regression models. Fifty-nine subjects completed 12 weeks of active treatment (Table 1).

Although SANS totals and sub-scores showed significant positive differences due to active treatment, the magnitude of clinical improvement due to drug treatment reflected by the impressive difference in CGI-I scores (0.46 units) did not seem to be accounted for by the relatively subtle positive changes seen in the SANS scores. Thus a variety of subgroup analyses were undertaken, and will be briefly discussed.

Given that selegiline has both antiparkinsonian and antidepressant properties, it might be objected that rather than specific effects on negative symptoms, what was observed were the drug's antiparkinsonian and antidepressant effects. However, a subgroup analysis comparing subjects with milder versus more severe baseline extrapyramidal symptoms, showed minimal effect on outcome, and there was no difference between drug and placebo in change in extrapyramidal symptoms. And although selegiline has been shown to have antidepressant properties, it is well established that selegiline's antidepressant properties are very limited at the MAO-B selective doses, as used in this study (Bodkin & Kwon, 2001). In addition, we had

Table 1. **Sample Description, Baseline Measures and Treatment Response**

CHARACTERISTICS[a]	SELEGILINE		PLACEBO		χ^2 OR t[b]	p
Subjects	33	100	34	100	–	–
Females	5	14.7	6	17.1	0.08	0.82
Caucasian	29	85.3	28	80.0	0.34	0.56
Employed	4	12.1	6	17.1	0.34	0.56
Age at baseline	38.0	9.0	39.9	8.7	0.90	0.37
Age at onset	23.1	9.4	24.6	7.3	0.72	0.47
Neuroleptic dosage (CPZ-eqv)	727	737	570	476	1.03	0.31

	BASELINE		ENDPOINT			
SYMPTOM RATINGS[c]	SELEGILINE	PLACEBO	SELEGILINE	PLACEBO	z[d]	p
1. SANS affective flattening	3.48 1.03	3.53 0.71	2.78 1.14	3.00 1.10	1.15	0.25
2. SANS avolition/ apathy	3.64 0.74	3.68 0.68	2.82 1.04	3.15 0.96	2.63	0.009
3. SANS alogia	2.94 1.29	2.79 1.09	2.06 1.22	2.29 1.27	0.20	0.84
4. SANS anhedonia	3.85 0.57	3.85 0.66	3.33 0.82	3.56 0.99	2.15	0.032
5. SANS attention	2.48 1.39	2.38 1.16	1.79 1.32	1.85 1.26	0.74	0.46
6. SANS total	16.4 3.69	16.2 3.15	12.8 3.71	13.9 4.15	1.98	0.048
8. BPRS thought disturbance	7.27 3.25	7.26 3.32	6.94 2.90	7.06 2.90	0.05	0.96
9. BPRS total score	41.4 9.70	40.8 10.1	37.2 8.80	40.4 10.4	2.47	0.014
10. CGI-S scale	4.48 0.91	4.34 0.94	4.42 0.94	4.47 0.86	3.13	0.002
11. CGI-I[e]	– –	– –	3.30 1.33	3.76 1.13	3.71	<0.001
12. SAEPS total	3.79 2.83	3.47 2.42	2.91 3.20	2.91 2.85	1.00	0.32
13. HDRS total	15.6 6.89	18.3 7.38	13.1 6.36	16.6 8.13	1.86	0.064

SAEPS: Simpson–Angus Ratings EPS scale.
[a] Table entries are n, % for nominal measures and mean, SD for continuous measures.
[b] Degrees of freedom = 1 for χ^2 used with nominal measures and 65 for t-statistics for continuous measures.
[c] On all scales, larger values indicate greater symptom severity.
[d] z-statistics and p-values are based on panel data random effects regression methods, with change-from-baseline as the outcome variable. At baseline and endpoint, selegiline and placebo Ns were 33/34 and 28/32, respectively.
[e] CGI-I consists of change-from-prior measurement data, so no baseline values are available.

excluded from the study patients requiring antidepressant medication or with diagnoses of mood disorders. Furthermore, the differential changes seen in the HDRS were largely attributable to the functional impairment item No. 7, rather than specific symptoms of depressive illness. In fact, the only specific difference favoring placebo treated subjects in the entire study was in severity of guilt as measured by the HDRS item No. 2.

Interestingly, although depressive symptom severity did not differ significantly between treatment groups, mood state was quite specifically impacted by drug treatment. The wide range of emotions constituting subjective mood state has been factor-analyzed into two independent factors – positive affect, comprising such feelings as cheerfulness, enthusiasm and enjoyment; and negative affect, comprising various states of distress – such as fear, anger, and dismay (Gray, 1991; Watson *et al.*, 1988). At each study visit, we administered the Positive and Negative

Affect Scale (PANAS), a psychometrically robust scale developed to measure these two aspects of emotion (Watson *et al.*, 1988). Although subjective mood state is highly variable, and quite difficult to measure reliably, we succeeded in finding a specific difference between study groups. For subjects completing the 12-week study, positive affect, as measured by the PANAS, increased 11.0% for selegiline-treated subjects, and decreased 3.1% for subjects receiving placebo ($p = 0.04$). However, negative affect did not differ at all between groups. As Jeffrey Gray has elucidated (Gray, 1991), activation of specific dopaminergic pathways underlies positive affect, but has little or no relation to negative affect. Thus the specific mood changes observed with selegiline treatment were consistent with the drug's mechanism of action. Perhaps because of this mood-brightening effect, virtually all study subjects elected to remain on selegiline after completion of the trial.

In an attempt to more fully characterize the effects of selegiline on negative symptoms, we conducted exploratory analyses, and found that relative to placebo controls, selegiline treated subjects experienced reduced thought disorder (BPRS "conceptual disorganization") and restlessness (BPRS "tension and activation"), increased engagement in activities (HDRS "Work and activities"), as well as relative worsening of guilt (HDRS "guilt"). The first three of these changes are consistent with stimulant-like effects of active treatment. The reported worsening of guilt may also suggest a cognitive effect, reflecting study subjects' increased sensitivity to their state and their surroundings.

Comparing subgroups of study subjects with differing baseline characteristics, we found that subjects demonstrating greatest improvement were receiving high doses of neuroleptics and exhibited the least positive symptoms at baseline. No treatment effects were seen in patients receiving doses less than 400 chlorpromazine equivalents daily, and almost none were observed in patients displaying significant florid psychotic symptoms. This may support a hypothesis that selegiline serves as an antidote to excessive dopamine receptor blockade by antipsychotic medication, manifested by symptoms more subtle than gross EPS; alternatively it may indicate that at higher doses of medication, florid symptoms in this quite ill population were better controlled, making changes in negative symptoms more discernable.

Several subgroup analyses showed no clinically significant differences in treatment response according to baseline characteristics, for example, baseline depressive symptom severity, negative symptom severity, and extrapyramidal symptom severity. However, the comparison between robust responders to drug versus robust responders to placebo seems to reveal an important feature of selegiline's specific effects. The two groups only differed significantly in BPRS conceptual disorganization. Robust responders to the study drug demonstrated a 36.7% ($n = 10$) improvement in conceptual disorganization and robust responders to placebo demonstrated a 16.7% ($n = 4$) worsening in the category ($p = 0.04$). Improvement in mental organization may underlie global functional improvement.

A surprisingly powerful predictor of clinical benefit from selegiline was baseline cigarette smoking status. When divided into smokers and non-smokers, the drug/placebo separation was dramatically greater among smokers. Interestingly, there is similar published evidence regarding another effective remedy for negative symptoms, clozapine. For example, in one study, smokers exhibited greater treatment response to clozapine than non-smokers and clozapine treatment was associated with a decrease in smoking, suggesting that clozapine treatment may in some way reduce the need for smoking (McEvoy *et al.*, 1999). These findings appear to suggest that one of the reasons for the well established elevated rate of smoking in patients with chronic schizophrenia (McEvoy *et al.*, 1999) may be to ameliorate the hypo-dopaminergic state that underlie negative symptoms. Thus, in the present study, the population of smokers may be "self-selected" for those negative symptoms that selegiline appears to remedy.

Unique Aspects of Trial

The present study provided much more conclusive findings than prior controlled trials. It utilized a sufficient N and a long enough period of experimental treatment to differentiate drug effect from placebo effect. Also enough clinical data was gathered to offer some preliminary insight into the specific, finer grain clinical characteristics of the drug's therapeutic effects.

Conclusions

Attention to the therapeutics of negative symptoms is a relatively new area in schizophrenia research. Selegiline therapy in the chronically medicated psychotic patient potentially dovetails with the dramatic move away from neuroleptics and toward so-called atypical antipsychotic drugs. Both approaches to limit the inhibition of dopaminergic pathways in a clinical population that, since the discovery of chlorpromazine, has suffered from the adverse consequences of central nervous system (CNS) dopamine blockade, which include impairment of the function of midbrain reward pathways and prefrontal executive function. The next step in clinical investigation should be to explore the effect of concomitant therapy with selegiline and atypical antipsychotic agent, which may offer a yet superior approach to the clinical management of negative symptomatology.

Translation to Clinical Practice

Concomitant selegiline should be introduced only after antipsychotic dosage is optimized to provide adequate suppression of positive symptoms while minimizing the behavioral toxicities that contribute to negative symptoms. In patients who still present with significant negative symptomatology, assessment should be made for underlying depressive illness, which should be treated conventionally. In those patients who manifest a burden of negative symptoms and do not require or do not benefit from antidepressant treatment, selegiline may be introduced at 5 mg bid.

Summary of How to Treat Negative Symptoms Incorporating the Results of This Data

In cases of schizophrenia marked by significant negative, low-dose selegiline may be prescribed in addition to ongoing antipsychotic therapy. Therapeutic effects may be subtle and be slow to emerge, so a careful baseline assessment of the severity of negative symptoms is recommended, with re-evaluation at several-month intervals.

It cannot be recommended on the basis of these findings to increase selegiline dose beyond the MAO-B selective dosage range (5–15 mg/day) because of the risk of hypertensive crisis in a population ill-suited to follow complex dietary restrictions.

References

Adan, F., & Siris, S.G. (1989). Trials of adjunctive alprazolam in negative symptom patients. *Canadian Journal of Psychiatry*, 34, 326–328.

Amsterdam, J.D. (2003). A double-blind, placebo-controlled trial of the safety and efficacy of selegiline transdermal system without dietary restrictions in patients with major depressive disorder. *Journal of Clinical Psychiatry*, 64, 208–214.

Andreasen, N.C. (1982). Negative symptoms in schizophrenia: definition and reliability. *Archives of General Psychiatry*, 39,784–788.

Ayd, F.J., & Blackwell, B. (eds.) (1970). *Discoveries in Biological Psychiatry*. Philadelphia: Lippincott.

Bermanzohn, P.C., & Siris, S.G. (1992). Akinesia: a syndrome common to parkinsonism, retarded depression, and negative symptoms of schizophrenia. *Comprehensive Psychiatry*, 33, 221–232.

Bodkin, J.A. (1990). Emerging uses for high-potency benzodiazepines in psychotic disorders. *Journal of Clinical Psychiatry*, 55 (Suppl.), 41–46.

Bodkin, J.A., & Amsterdam, J.D. (2002). Transdermal selegiline in major depression: a double-blind, placebo-controlled study in outpatients. *American Journal of Psychiatry*, 195, 1869–1875.

Bodkin, J.A., & Kwon, A.E. (2001). Selegiline and other atypical monoamine oxidase inhibitors in depression. *Psychiatric Annals*, 31, 385–391.

Bodkin, J.A., Cohen, B.M., Solomon, M.S., Cannon, S.E., Zornberg, G.L., & Cole, J.O. (1996). Treatment of negative symptoms in schizophrenia and schizoaffective disorder by selegiline augmentation of antipsychotic medication. *The Journal of Nervous and Mental Disease*, 184, 295–301.

Bodkin, J.A, Siris, S.G., Bermanzohn, P.C., Hennen, J., & Cole, J.O. (2005). Treating negative symptoms of schizophrenic outpatients by selegiline augmentation of antipsychotic medication: a multi-center, double-blind, placebo-controlled trial. *American Journal of Psychiatry*, 162, 388–390.

Bucci, L. (1987). The negative symptoms of schizophrenia and the monoamine oxidase inhibitors. *Psychopharmacology*, 91, 104–108.

Carpenter, W.T., Heinrichs, D.W., Wagman, A.M., & Althea, M.I. (1988). Deficit and nondeficit forms of schizophrenia: the concept. *American Journal of Psychiatry*, 145, 578–583.

Cole, J.O., Jones, R.T., & Klerman, G.L. (1961). Drug therapy. *Progress in Neurology and Psychiatry*, 16, 539–574.

Davis, K.L., Kahn, R.S., Ko, G., & Davidson, M. (1991). Dopamine in schizophrenia: a review and reconceptualization. *American Journal of Psychiatry*, 148, 1474–1486.

Goff, D.C., Renshaw, P.F., Sarid-Segal, O., Dreyfus, D., Amico, E.T., & Ciraulo, D.A. (1993). A placebo-controlled trial of selegiline (L-deprenyl) in the treatment of tardive dyskinesia. *Biological Psychiatry*, 33, 700–706.

Goff, D.C., Midha, K.K., Sarid-Segal, O., Hubbard, J.W., & Amico, E.T. (1995). A placebo-controlled trial of fluoxetine added to neuroleptic in patients with schizophrenia. *Psychopharmacology*, 117, 417–423.

Gray, J.A. (1991). Neural systems, emotion and personality. In: Madden, J. (ed.), *Neurobiology of Learning, Emotion and Affect*. New York: Raven Press, pp. 273–306.

Gupta, S., Droney, T., Kyser, A., & Keller, P. (1999). Selegiline augmentation of antipsychotics for the treatment of negative symptoms in schizophrenia. *Comprehensive Psychiatry*, 40, 148–150.

Jungerman, T., Rabinowitz, D., & Klein, E. (1999). Deprenyl augmentation for treating negative symptoms of schizophrenia: a double-blind, controlled study. *Journal of Clinical Psychopharmacology*, 19, 522–525.

Kamman, G.R., Freeman, J.G., & Lucero, R. (1953). The effect of iproniazid on the behavior of long-term mental patients. *Journal of Nervous and Mental Disease*, 118, 391–407.

Kane, J., Honigfeld, G., Singer, J., & Meltzer, H.Y. (1988). Clozapine for the treatment-resistant schizophrenic. A double-blind comparison with chlorpromazine. *Archives of General Psychiatry*, 45, 789–796.

Klein, D.F., Gittelman, R., Quitkin, F., & Rifkin, A. (1980). *Diagnosis and Drug Treatment of Psychiatric Disorders: adults and Children* (2nd ed.). Baltimore, MD: Williams & Wilkins.

Knoll, J. (1983). Deprenyl (selegiline): the history of its development and pharmacological action. *Acta Neurologica Scandinavia*, 95 (Suppl.), 57–80.

Lees, A. (1991). Selegiline hydrochloride and cognition. *Acta Neurologica Scandanavia*, 136 (Suppl.), 91–94.

Levi-Minzi, S., Bermanzohn, P.C., & Siris, S.G. (1991). Bromocriptine for "negative" schizophrenia. *Comprehensive Psychiatry*, 32, 210–216.

Mandel, S., Grunblatt, E., Riederer, P., Gerlach, M., Levites, Y., & Youdim, M.B. (2003). Neuroprotective strategies in Parkinson's disease: an update on progress. *CNS Drugs*, 17(10), 729–762.

Mann, J.J., Aarons, S.F., Wilner, P.J., Keilp, J.G., Sweeney, J.A., Pearlstein, T., Francis, A.J., Kocsis, J.H., & Brown, R.P. (1989). A controlled study of the antidepressant efficacy and side effects of (-)-deprenyl. A selective monoamine oxidase inhibitor. *Archives of General Psychiatry*, 46, 45–50.

McEvoy, J.P., Freudenreich, O., & Wilson, W.H. (1999). Smoking and therapeutic response to clozapine in patients with schizophrenia. *Biological Psychiatry*, 46, 125–129.

Perenyi, A., Goswami, U., Frecska, E., Arato, M., & Bela, A. (1991). L-deprenyl in treating negative symptoms of schizophrenia. *Psychiatry Research*, 42, 188–191.

Rifkin, A., Quitkin, F., & Klein, D.F. (1975). Akinesia: a poorly recognized drug-induced extrapyramidal disorder. *Archives of General Psychiatry*, 32, 672–675.

Silver, H., & Nassar, A. (1992). Fluvoxamine improves negative symptoms in treated chronic schizophrenia: an add-on double-blind, placebo-controlled study. *Biological Psychiatry*, 31, 698–704.

Siris, S.G., van Kammen, D.P., & Docherty, J.P. (1978). The use of anti-depressant medications in schizophrenia: a review of the literature. *Archives of General Psychiatry*, 35, 1368–1377.

Tetrud, J.W., & Langston, J.W. (1989). The effect of Deprenyl (Selegiline) on the natural history of Parkinson's disease. *Science*, 245, 519–522.

Watson, D., Clark, L.A., & Tellegen, A. (1988). Development and validation of brief measures of positive and negative affect: the PANAS scales. *Journal of Personality and Social Psychology*, 54, 1063–1070.

Wirshing, D.A. (2001). Adverse effects of atypical antipsychotics. *Journal of Clinical Psychiatry*, 62 (Suppl.), 7–10.

Progress in Neurotherapeutics and Neuropsychopharmacology, 1:1, 133–147 © 2006 Cambridge University Press
DOI: 10.1017/S1748232105000133   Printed in the United Kingdom

Analysis of the Cognitive Enhancing Effects of Modafinil in Schizophrenia

Danielle C. Turner and Barbara J. Sahakian

Department of Psychiatry, University of Cambridge, Addenbrooke's Hospital, Cambridge, UK;
Email: dct23@cam.ac.uk; jenny.hall@cambsmh.nhs.uk

Key words: schizophrenia; modafinil; Provigil; smart drugs; cognitive enhancement; high functioning.

Introduction and Overview

Numerous neuropsychiatric disorders, such as attention deficit hyperactivity disorder (ADHD), schizophrenia, frontotemporal dementia and Parkinson's disease, are characterized by cognitive impairments. The potential public health benefit of improving current treatments for cognitive disabilities is undisputed (Meltzer, 2003). The disorder of schizophrenia illustrates particularly well the need for specific treatments of cognitive dysfunction. The clinical targets for schizophrenia have traditionally been the delusions and hallucinations that characterize the disorder, and for which neuroleptic agents are most efficacious (Campbell *et al.*, 1999). However, although these symptoms define the core *diagnostic* criteria of this illness, it is now recognized that the cognitive and motivational impairments in schizophrenia are closely related to the profound long-term disability typically produced by the disease (Hyman & Fenton, 2003). Indeed, cognitive deficits are the major cause of poor psychosocial function and impoverished quality of life in patients with schizophrenia for whom psychosis is controlled by currently available therapies (Geyer & Tamminga, 2004).

Neuropsychological studies of patients with schizophrenia have consistently identified deficits on tests of executive function, known to be sensitive to frontal lobe damage. Deficits in cognitive flexibility, working memory and planning have been widely reported, together with more recent evidence of impairments in inhibitory control (Badcock *et al.*, 2002; Pantelis *et al.*, 1999; Elliott *et al.*, 1995; Pantelis & Brewer, 1995). Moreover, cognitive flexibility, as measured by the

Correspondence should be addressed to: Dr Danielle C. Turner, Department of Psychiatry, University of Cambridge, Box 189, Addenbrooke's Hospital, Cambridge, CB2 2QQ, Ph: +1223 245 151; Email: dct23@cam.ac.uk.

Wisconsin Card Sorting Test (WCST), has been related to community outcome in these patients (Hartman *et al.*, 2003; Koren *et al.*, 1998; Green, 1996) and to response to psychological intervention (Wykes *et al.*, 2003).

Stimulant medication is known to enhance cognitive function in healthy volunteers (Elliott *et al.*, 1997). It has also been used previously in the treatment of schizophrenia, most commonly in an attempt to treat patients with prominent negative symptoms (Angrist *et al.*, 1982). However, studies have reported a re-emergence or worsening of positive symptoms as a result of the dopaminergic activity of these drugs (Szeszko *et al.*, 1999; Levy *et al.*, 1993). Nevertheless, circumstantial evidence has accumulated to suggest that stimulant treatment might be of benefit to cognitive and negative symptoms in patients with schizophrenia (Davidson & Keefe, 1995; Carpenter *et al.*, 1992; Goldberg *et al.*, 1991). Modafinil, a non-dopaminergic stimulant, was therefore considered as a potential agent for use in schizophrenia. Modafinil is a novel wake-promoting agent that is known to have significant cognitive enhancing effects in young healthy adults (Muller *et al.*, 2004; Turner *et al.*, 2003b), older adults (Randall *et al.*, 2004) and adult patients with ADHD (Turner *et al.*, 2004a), possibly through a mechanism involving reduced cognitive impulsivity.

Purpose of the Trial

The present study sought to examine the potential of modafinil as a cognitive enhancer in chronic, stable, high-functioning patients with schizophrenia. Given that traditional (dopaminergic) stimulants appear to have some beneficial effects in schizophrenia (Davidson & Keefe, 1995), but with the unavoidable exacerbation of positive symptoms (Levy *et al.*, 1993), it was hypothesized that modafinil, with its reduced dopaminergic activity, might be more appropriate for use in schizophrenia.

Agent

Relevant Past Clinical Experience, Phase I or Preclinical Data

Modafinil (Provigil™), a novel wake-promoting agent, was licensed in the UK for the treatment of narcolepsy in 1997 (Provigil, 1997). Modafinil is particularly known for its ability to potently increase waking in animals and humans, with less peripheral (e.g. cardiovascular) or central side-effects and abuse potential than amphetamine (Jasinski, 2000). The precise mode of action of modafinil remains unknown. The most striking difference between conventional stimulants, such as amphetamine, and modafinil is that modafinil appears to produce arousal through a mechanism that does not directly stimulate the dopaminergic system at therapeutic doses (Taylor & Russo, 2000; Ferraro *et al.*, 1997; Lin *et al.*, 1996, 1992, but see

Wisor & Eriksson, 2005; Wisor *et al.*, 2001). Modafinil, unlike amphetamine, does not stimulate the release of dopamine from preloaded synaptosomes (Simon *et al.*, 1994), has no anxiogenic effects (Simon *et al.*, 1994), and does not induce stereotypy in rats (Duteil *et al.*, 1990). The low abuse potential of modafinil also suggests a non-dopaminergic pathway activity (Jasinski, 2000), and likely treatment benefits over stimulants such as methylphenidate. There are suggestions that the wake-promoting effects of modafinil may require an intact noradrenergic system (Lin *et al.*, 1992), although other authors have argued against a noradrenergic mechanism of action (Shelton *et al.*, 1995; Akaoka *et al.*, 1991). Most recently, it has been suggested that the noradrenergic projections from the locus coeruleus to the forebrain are not necessary for the wakefulness-promoting action of modafinil, although modafinil's effects on wakefulness can be attenuated by the adrenergic antagonism (Wisor & Eriksson, 2005). It has also been postulated that a catecholaminergic tone, particularly in the cortical noradrenergic neurones, is required for modafinil to exert a serotonin-mediated inhibition, or reduction, of γ-amino-*n*-butyric acid (GABA) release in the cerebral cortex (Tanganelli *et al.*, 1995, 1994). Recent evidence has suggested that modafinil might possibly also be acting via a mechanism that is similar to the newly discovered neuropeptides orexin-A and -B (Scammell *et al.*, 2000; Chemelli *et al.*, 1999), which are central to canine models of narcolepsy, to promote histamine release (Ishizuka *et al.*, 2003).

Prior to our study (Turner *et al.*, 2004b) there were no well-controlled studies using modafinil in schizophrenia. Two case studies had suggested some improvements in negative symptomatology with modafinil (Yu *et al.*, 2002) and modafinil had also been shown to improve antipsychotic-associated sedation in three patients with schizophrenia (Makela *et al.*, 2003). This study was therefore of great interest in terms of modafinil's potential as a cognitive enhancer in schizophrenia.

Clinical Trial

Subjects

Twenty high-functioning adult patients (16 male, 4 female) meeting criteria for a DSM-IV diagnosis of schizophrenia (American Psychiatric Association, 1994) were recruited from the Cambridge Psychiatric Rehabilitation Service. Patients had a mean age of 43 ± 9 years (range 26–59 years), an average NART verbal IQ (as indexed by the National Adult Reading Test, Nelson, 1982) of 110 ± 6 (range 100–126) and had been in formal education for an average of 13 ± 2 years (range 10–16 years). The study was approved by the Cambridge Local Research Ethics Committee and written informed consent was given by all patients prior to testing.

All patients were in a stable clinical condition, living either independently or in sheltered accommodation with support, and on stabilized doses of neuroleptic medication. Eighteen patients were stabilized on clozapine (range 100–600 mg/day), one on olanzapine (10 mg/day) and one patient received a twice-monthly depot injection of pipotiazine (75 mg). In addition, all had a Mini Mental State Examination (MMSE) (Folstein *et al.*, 1975) score of ≥26 to exclude marked overall intellectual impairment. The mean Global Assessment Scale score (which ranges from 0 to 100) (Luborsky, 1962) for the group was 40.7 ± 7.12 (range 31–62), indicative of patients with "major impairment in several areas, such as work, family relations, judgement, thinking or mood". Patients were also assessed using the Comprehensive Assessment of Symptoms and History scale (Andreasen *et al.*, 1992) (readers are directed to the original paper for full details, Turner *et al.*, 2004b). Mean duration of illness, from first admission to a psychiatric facility, was 17.3 ± 9.7 years (range 4–39 years). Exclusion criteria included any significant motor or visual impairment, the concurrent use of any medication contraindicated with modafinil or an NART verbal IQ score of <90.

Trial Methods

A randomized double-blind, placebo-controlled, crossover design was used, with 10 participants randomized to receive a single oral dose of a lactose placebo on the first session followed by 200 mg modafinil in the second session (the P/D group) and 10 participants randomized to receive drug first, followed by placebo (the D/P group). Both groups were matched for age, NART verbal IQ and education level ($F(1,18) \leq 0.80$, $p \geq 0.382$). For each patient, testing sessions were separated by at least a week.

Instruments/Measures

PSYCHOLOGICAL MEASURES
Patients were tested on a comprehensive neuropsychological test battery including tests from the CANTAB (www.camcog.com). The tests used were the same as those used in our previous studies with modafinil (Turner *et al.*, 2004a, 2003b) although the battery was shortened to increase patient compliance. Where available, parallel versions of the tasks were used to limit practice effects. The order in which patients received the tasks differed for the placebo and drug conditions, and was randomized across patients. All computerized tasks were run on an Advantech personal computer (Model PPC-120T-RT), and responses registered either via the touch-sensitive screen or a button box, depending on the task. A brief description of the key measures for each of the tasks is presented in Table 1.

PHYSIOLOGICAL MEASURES
Blood pressure and pulse measurements were taken using a Criticare Systems Inc. Comfort Cuff™ (Model 507NJ) at four time points: before drug administration, immediately prior to testing (2 hours post-drug), 1 hour into testing (3 hours post-drug) and on completion of the study (4 hours post-drug).

Table 1. **Summary of Neuropsychological Tests**

TASK	DESCRIPTION	IMPORTANT MEASURES
Computerized tasks – attentional battery		
IDED	Discrimination learning, testing the ability to selectively attend to and set shift between shape, colour or number stimulus dimensions	Total errors Total reversal errors Total EDS errors
Computerized tasks – planning and working memory battery		
NTOL	A spatial planning test, involving planning a sequence of moves to achieve a goal arrangement of coloured balls without moving the balls	Mean attempts Latency (ms)
SWM[a]	A test of spatial working memory and strategy performance to find individually hidden "blue tokens" without returning to a box where one has previously been found	Strategy score Total between errors (*returning to a box where a token has been found*) Total within errors (*returning to a box that has already been inspected*)
SSP[a]	A test of spatial memory span to recall the order in which a series of boxes were highlighted	Span length Total errors
Computerized tasks – response inhibition		
STOP	A test of response inhibition. Patients make speeded left or right responses on "go" trials but withhold their response on "stop" trials (signalled by a 300-Hz tone). Race model allows estimation of the time taken to internally suppress a "go" response (SSRT)	Go reaction time (ms) SSRT (*a measure of response inhibition*) Errors (*incorrect discrimination responses on "go" trials*)
Verbal task		
Digit span	A test of short-term digit memory, taken from the Wechsler Adult Intelligence Scale. Two digit sequences of the same length are presented at each stage	Forwards score Backwards score *Both calculated as the total number of correct digit sequences achieved*
Computerized tasks – visual memory battery		
PRM[a]	A two-choice test of abstract visual pattern recognition memory	Percentage correct Response latency (ms)
DMTS[a]	A four-choice test of simultaneous and delayed matching to sample of abstract patterns, which share colour or pattern with the distractors	Percentage correct Latency (ms)

IDED: Intradimensional-extradimensional attentional set shifting task; EDS: extradimensional shift stage of the IDED task; NTOL: "One-Touch" Tower of London Spatial planning task; SWM: spatial working memory test; SSP: spatial span test; STOP: stop-signal reaction time (SSRT) task; PRM: pattern recognition memory test; DMTS: delayed matching to sample test. [a]: indicates tasks taken from the CANTAB battery. Adapted from Turner *et al.* (2004b).

SUBJECTIVE MEASURES

Patients were asked to complete visual analogue scales (Bond & Lader, 1974) before administration of the drug and at three intervals during the testing session: immediately prior to testing, 1 hour into testing and on completion of testing. At each of the four time points patients were asked to rate their feelings in terms of 16 well-validated dimensions (Turner *et al.*, 2004a, 2003a, b).

Primary and Secondary Outcomes

The primary outcome measure for this study was cognitive response to modafinil, assessed using a battery of eight well-validated cognitive tests. Secondary outcome measures were physiological function (assessed in terms of blood pressure and heart rate) and subjective effects (measured using visual analogue scales).

Analysis

To investigate the effect of experimental treatment upon test performance, repeated-measures analysis of variance (ANOVA) with drug (drug or placebo) as the within-subjects factor and order (P/D or D/P) as the between-subjects factor, with an additional within-subjects factor of level or difficulty if appropriate, was used. Where appropriate, the Wilcoxon signed-rank test was used for non-parametric data. Crossover designs have the potential problem that practice may confound the interpretation of drug effects. We attempted to reduce practice effects wherever possible by using parallel versions of the tasks. However, in instances where significant drug $\times$ order interactions or main effects of order were identified, we felt it was of interest to explore the between-subjects effects on the first or second sessions alone, despite the reduced power (only 10 patients in each group). Between-group means (or median for reaction time on the stop-signal reaction time task, STOP) for single scores were analysed using a one-way ANOVA, or the equivalent Kruskal–Wallis test. Where several readings were taken for the same score, a repeated-measures ANOVA was used.

As the motivation for this study was to determine the overall cognitive profile of modafinil in schizophrenia, our interest lay equally in ascertaining the lack of an effect on particular variables, as in identifying the presence of a significant group difference on other variables. The former conclusion of a lack of effect is subject to Type II errors and the latter, the presence of an effect, to Type I errors (Howell, 1997). Taking this into consideration, we took $p > 0.1$ in reporting "no effect" and $p < 0.05$ in reporting "an effect".

Results

EFFICACY

The main results for this study are summarized in Table 2 (for more details readers are directed to the original paper, Turner *et al.*, 2004b). The results of this study demonstrate that, in high-functioning patients with schizophrenia, modafinil is associated with a specific pattern of cognitive enhancement. The most striking improvements were on attentional set shifting (cognitive flexibility) and verbal memory. Patients on modafinil passed significantly more stages of the IDED attentional set shifting task and made significantly fewer errors at the crucial, and most difficult, extradimensional stage of this task (Figure 1). This improvement

Table 2. **Summary of Test Results**

	MEAN ± STANDARD DEVIATION		MAIN EFFECT OF DRUG
	PLACEBO	DRUG	*P*-VALUE
IDED			
Total errors	42.60 ± 31.34	35.55 ± 25.31	0.261
Total reversal errors	14.40 ± 11.70	16.35 ± 12.10	0.382
Total EDS errors	13.65 ± 10.69	8.60 ± 7.35	0.039
NTOL			
Mean attempts (all moves)	10.47 ± 2.74	9.67 ± 2.24	0.072
Latency (all moves) (ms)	14883 ± 5113	19874 ± 8547	0.003
SWM			
Strategy score	35.70 ± 7.75	34.90 ± 7.28	0.424
Between errors	40.35 ± 26.89	42.60 ± 26.23	0.593
Within errors	3.05 ± 3.44	4.50 ± 5.53	0.191
SSP			
Span length	4.95 ± 1.43	5.15 ± 1.57	0.276
Total errors	80.70 ± 27.78	80.85 ± 28.98	0.955
STOP			
Go reaction time (ms)	567.21 ± 201.76	565.21 ± 160.62	0.793
SSRT (ms)	193.66 ± 75.92	187.45 ± 41.49	0.506
Discrimination errors	4.47 ± 4.72	3.42 ± 3.81	0.160
Digit span			
Forwards score	7.70 ± 2.66	8.80 ± 2.97	0.018
Backwards score	6.05 ± 2.96	6.85 ± 2.96	0.006
PRM			
Percentage correct (immediate)	80.83 ± 12.42	81.45 ± 12.49	0.803
Response latency (immediate) (ms)	2336 ± 722	2255 ± 826	0.445
Percentage correct (delayed)	7.92 ± 15.82	72.92 ± 14.08	0.097
Response latency (delayed) (ms)	2225 ± 991	2486 ± 1092	0.116
DMTS			
Percentage correct	66.33 ± 20.57	65.00 ± 20.51	0.845
Latency (ms)	4692 ± 2048	4930 ± 1736	0.734

Values shown for each variable are the mean and standard deviation for each group. For abbreviations with expansions refer to footnotes of Table 1. Adapted from Turner *et al.* (2004b).

appears specific to schizophrenia as similar changes were not seen in our other studies (Turner *et al.*, 2004a, 2003b).

Modafinil also significantly improved performance on tests of verbal memory, with clear improvements seen on both forward and backward digit span. Similarly, trends towards improvements in visual memory (delayed pattern recognition memory) and spatial planning (NTOL, One-Touch Tower of London test of planning) were seen following modafinil. Performance on these two latter tests is significantly improved by modafinil in healthy adults and patients with ADHD (Turner *et al.*, 2004a, 2003b), indicating modafinil's consistent ability to modulate these cognitive functions. Similarly, as in our other studies (Turner *et al.*, 2004a, 2003b), a slowing in latency with modafinil on the spatial planning task was

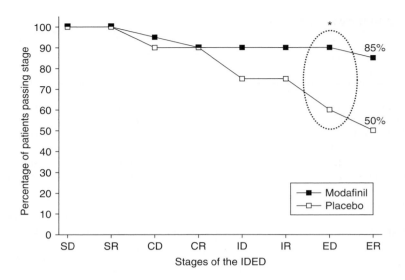

Fig. 1.
Modafinil significantly improves cognitive flexibility.
Patients receiving modafinil performed significantly better at the IDED attentional set shifting task than when receiving placebo (50% completed the task on placebo, 85% on modafinil; $\chi^2 = 5.58$, df = 1, $p < 0.025$). In particular, significantly more patients passed the extradimensional stage of the task on modafinil ($\chi^2 = 3.96$, df = 1, $p < 0.05$) as indicated by the dotted circle (*). This is a critical stage of the task that resembles the set shift in the WCST. The stages of the task are SD (simple discrimination), SR (simple reversal), CD (compound discrimination), CR (compound reversal), ID (intradimensional shift), IR (intradimensional reversal), ED (extradimensional shift), ER (extradimensional reversal). Adapted from Turner *et al.* (2004b).

observed in patients with schizophrenia. This slowing does not appear to be a simple psychomotor effect of drug, as standard reaction time (measured by the median "go" reaction time on the STOP) was unaffected by modafinil.

TOLERABILITY
Subjectively, patients did not record any significant effect of modafinil according to the visual analogue scales ($p > 0.1$). However, it is possible that this was due to a lack of insight by the patients into their changing mood as two patients volunteered information suggesting that they experienced some subjective changes to modafinil. The patients in this study also showed no main effect of modafinil on systolic blood pressure, diastolic blood pressure or pulse, although when receiving drug, the group did show a more fluctuating systolic blood pressure over the testing session compared to when on placebo ($F(3,54) = 2.81, p = 0.048$).

SAFETY
No patients experienced any adverse events in our study. However this was a single-dose study using a moderate dose of modafinil and additional studies must be

performed to assess the tolerability of modafinil in more long-term studies. Additionally, participants in our study were highly selected to maximize the detection of any cognitive effect of modafinil. Only patients in whom the positive and negative symptoms had been stable for extended periods of time, and who were expected to remain stable for the duration of the study were included. The majority of patients (18/20) were on clozapine.

Our study used a single 200 mg dose of modafinil, in agreement with previous dose-related work from our laboratory (Turner *et al.*, 2003b), and no adverse effects were noted (Turner *et al.*, 2004b). However, there have been some recent reports of modafinil being associated with an exacerbation of psychosis in patients with schizophrenia, and thus it is important that modafinil be used with caution in studies of patients with schizophrenia at this early stage. In one case report, a patient with schizophrenia became agitated with extreme disorganization of speech, paranoid delusions and auditory hallucinations following 800 mg per day of modafinil (Narendran *et al.*, 2002). In a more recent imaging study of modafinil in schizophrenia, acute relapse of psychosis was noted in one patient 4 days after taking a single 100 mg dose of modafinil (Spence *et al.*, 2005), while another study has also reported a worsening of psychosis in one patient following 100 mg modafinil as part of a behavioural study (Sevy *et al.*, 2005).

Unique Aspects of Trial

This proof-of-concept study was the first cognitive appraisal of modafinil in schizophrenia, using a rigorous randomized double-blind, placebo-controlled, crossover design and a comprehensive battery of well-validated cognitive tasks. Importantly, it showed that modafinil has very promising neurocognitive enhancing effects in schizophrenia. These results are the first definitive demonstration of pharmacological improvement of a core cognitive deficit in schizophrenia and highlight the potential susceptibility of cognitive functions to pharmacological mediation in these patients.

Conclusions

This study provides important evidence of a cognitive enhancing effect of modafinil in schizophrenia. If these improvements with modafinil are confirmed with long-term administration studies, these findings will have clear relevance for clinical practice. This is particularly true given the strong evidence showing that certain cognitive deficits might be important determinants of functional outcome in patients with schizophrenia.

Further work is needed to extend our understanding of modafinil's effects in a wider range of patients with schizophrenia and to examine further the effects on cognitive flexibility. Deficits in attentional set shifting at the extradimensional shift stage of the IDED task (the stage that was improved by modafinil in our study), have been demonstrated in young, stabilized patients (Elliott *et al.*, 1995). However, more generalized cognitive deficits on this task are observed in more severely ill patients with schizophrenia (Pantelis *et al.*, 1999). These patients fail to "learn set" and are impaired at both set shifting and concept formation, with many of the effects appearing to be related to symptomatology (Pantelis *et al.*, 1999). It cannot be assumed that all patients will derive equal benefit from modafinil. Nonetheless, these results from a group of chronic, stable, high-functioning patients (Turner *et al.*, 2004b) are encouraging, indicating that at least some patients may experience improvements in cognition from modafinil. It is important, however, that these results are confirmed with long-term chronic administration studies. Although there is evidence that cognitive impairments are relatively stable over time (Heaton *et al.*, 2001; Wykes *et al.*, 2000), it is not clear that cognitive improvements would show similar consistency.

Nevertheless, even small improvements in cognition may be clinically relevant to schizophrenia. Changes in memory over 1 year have been correlated with changes in quality of life (Buchanan *et al.*, 1994), while a change in cognitive flexibility has been related to improvement in social functioning (Wykes *et al.*, 1999). Similarly, improvements in WCST performance have been associated with improved social competence, and improvements in verbal memory with increased acquisition of psychosocial skills (Spaulding *et al.*, 1999). It has been proposed that in younger patients, improvements in executive functions and planning equivalent to a change of just one category on the WCST (which is analogous to the IDED attentional set shifting task) could enable patients to organize themselves enough to live independently outside a psychiatric institution (Davidson & Keefe, 1995). Modafinil may therefore have potential as an important therapy for cognitive impairment in patients with schizophrenia, particularly because of its beneficial effects on attentional set shifting.

Influence on the Field

Other Recent Advances

Since the publication of our study (Turner *et al.*, 2004b), other institutions have initiated research projects to examine the effects of modafinil in schizophrenia. A recent study has shown that a single low dose of modafinil (100 mg) modulates anterior cingulate cortex function in patients with chronic schizophrenia and that activation in this area correlated with cognitive performance (Spence *et al.*, 2005). However, another recent study examining the effects of modafinil (100–200 mg) on fatigue, symptomatology and cognitive functioning found no significant effect of modafinil (although the authors acknowledge several limitations with their study including a relative lack of power) (Sevy *et al.*, 2005).

Encouragingly, several larger studies examining the effects of modafinil in schizophrenia are also underway. The University of California, San Diego, has indicated that an 8-week outpatient study is being conducted to examine the safety and effectiveness of modafinil in treating negative symptoms in schizophrenia: http://mentalhealth.ucsd.edu/trials/SCZ.php. In addition, the National Institute of Mental Health in the USA is recruiting for a large randomized, double-blind, placebo-controlled study examining the effects of modafinil on cognitive function in patients with schizophrenia and normal controls, based on catechol-*O*-methyltransferase (COMT) genotype: http://www.clinicaltrials.gov/ct/show/NCT00057707?order=1. Expected enrolment for this study is 180 participants and it will certainly provide a more definitive answer as to modafinil's efficacy in schizophrenia.

How the Trial Results Fit into the Emerging Treatment and Research Framework

Modafinil, in contrast to other stimulant drugs such as methylphenidate, appears to have more consistent cognitive effects across different population groups and to be more suitable for use in schizophrenia (although additional studies are required to determine whether certain patients might be susceptible to suffering a relapse of psychosis on modafinil). Modafinil may serve to improve performance accuracy by causing an increased tendency for study participants to evaluate problems before initiating a response. This evaluative effect accords with current theories of reflection, a conceptually different form of impulsivity, in which performance is impaired due to a deficit in utilizing all available information before making a decision (Evenden, 1999). It is too early to anticipate how modafinil might be incorporated into treatment frameworks. However, this work has important implications for research into cognitive enhancement. The mechanism of action of modafinil is still to be fully elucidated and there is great interest to establish modafinil's precise pharmacological actions and the implications this will have for our understanding of cognitive flexibility, planning and inhibitory control. Research work in these areas will contribute to our understanding of the neural mechanisms of cognition and will foster research into more specific cognitive enhancing agents for schizophrenia as well as many other neuropsychiatric conditions characterized by cognitive impairment.

Relevant Regulatory Issues

This was a small-scale, investigator-led, proof-of-concept study funded by a Wellcome Trust Programme Grant awarded to T.W. Robbins, B.J. Everitt, B.J. Sahakian and A.C. Roberts, and was completed within the MRC (UK) Centre for Behavioural and Clinical Neuroscience. At the time of the study, Danielle Turner was funded by a Research Studentship from the Medical Research Council of the UK. The aim of this research was to examine the cognitive effects of a single dose of modafinil and thus this study does not meet FDA requirements for the assessment of therapeutic efficacy of a drug. Additional longer-term studies are required to address this question.

Translation to Clinical Practice

Modafinil is not licensed for use in schizophrenia, and large long-term studies are required in order to determine whether it might prove a useful agent for clinical use in these patients and how it might be incorporated into clinical guidelines.

The research described was a proof-of-concept study to examine the cognitive effects of a single dose of modafinil in schizophrenia. Further work is needed to determine the full extent of the effects of modafinil in these patients and the best approach for establishing treatment algorithms. It is expected that modafinil will only be used as an adjunctive treatment to antipsychotic medication, as it does not have any antipsychotic properties itself.

Summary of How to Treat the Disorder Incorporating the Results of the New Trial Data

This research showed that modafinil has important cognitive enhancing properties in schizophrenia, following a single dose of drug. This work demonstrates that it is possible to selectively improve cognitive performance in chronic, stable, high-functioning patients using targeted cognitive enhancers. However, replication with larger, more long-term studies in high-functioning patients as well as extending to more heterogeneous groups of patients is required to establish if modafinil has consistent effects on cognition. This work (Turner *et al.*, 2004b) used neuropsychological tests to tap core cognitive functions in schizophrenia that are related to functional ability, and it is important that future studies similarly address these issues of cognition as related to functional outcome.

References

Akaoka, H., *et al.* (1991). Effect of modafinil and amphetamine on the rat catecholaminergic neuron activity. *Neuroscience Letters*, 123(1), 20–22.

American Psychiatric Association. (1994). *Diagnostic and Statistical Manual of Mental Disorders* (4th ed.). Washington, DC: American Psychiatric Press.

Andreasen, N.C., *et al.* (1992). The Comprehensive Assessment of Symptoms and History (CASH). An instrument for assessing diagnosis and psychopathology. *Archives of General Psychiatry*, 49(8), 615–623.

Angrist, B., *et al.* (1982). Partial improvement in negative schizophrenic symptoms after amphetamine. *Psychopharmacology (Berl)*, 78(2), 128–130.

Badcock, J.C., *et al.* (2002). Acts of control in schizophrenia: dissociating the components of inhibition. *Psychological Medicine*, 32(2), 287–297.

Bond, A., & Lader, M. (1974). The use of analogue scales in rating subjective feelings. *British Journal of Medical Psychology*, 47, 211–218.

Buchanan, R.W., *et al.* (1994). The comparative efficacy and long-term effect of clozapine treatment on neuropsychological test performance. *Biological Psychiatry*, 36(11), 717–725.

Campbell, M., *et al.* (1999). The use of atypical antipsychotics in the management of schizophrenia. *British Journal of Clinical Pharmacology*, 47(1), 13–22.

Carpenter, M.D., *et al.* (1992). Methylphenidate augmentation therapy in schizophrenia. *Journal of Clinical Psychopharmacology*, 12(4), 273–275.

Chemelli, R.M., *et al.* (1999). Narcolepsy in orexin knockout mice: molecular genetics of sleep regulation. *Cell*, 98(4), 437–451.

Davidson, M., & Keefe, R.S. (1995). Cognitive impairment as a target for pharmacological treatment in schizophrenia. *Schizophrenia Research*, 17(1), 123–129.

Duteil, J., *et al.* (1990). Central alpha 1-adrenergic stimulation in relation to the behaviour stimulating effect of modafinil; studies with experimental animals. *European Journal of Pharmacology*, 180(1), 49–58.

Elliott, R., *et al.* (1995). Neuropsychological evidence for frontostriatal dysfunction in schizophrenia. *Psychological Medicine*, 25(3), 619–630.

Elliott, R., *et al.* (1997). Effects of methylphenidate on spatial working memory and planning in healthy young adults. *Psychopharmacology (Berl)*, 131(2), 196–206.

Evenden, J.L. (1999). Varieties of impulsivity. *Psychopharmacology (Berl)*, 146(4), 348–361.

Ferraro, L., *et al.* (1997). Modafinil: an antinarcoleptic drug with a different neurochemical profile to D-amphetamine and dopamine uptake blockers. *Biological Psychiatry*, 42(12), 1181–1183.

Folstein, M.F., *et al.* (1975). Mini-mental state. A practical method for grading the cognitive state of patients for the clinician. *Journal of Psychiatric Research*, 12(3), 189–198.

Geyer, M.A., & Tamminga, C.A. (2004). Measurement and treatment research to improve cognition in schizophrenia: neuropharmacological aspects. *Psychopharmacology*, 174(1), 1–2.

Goldberg, T.E., *et al.* (1991). Cognitive and behavioral effects of the coadministration of dextroamphetamine and haloperidol in schizophrenia. *American Journal of Psychiatry*, 148(1), 78–84.

Green, M.F. (1996). What are the functional consequences of neurocognitive deficits in schizophrenia? *American Journal of Psychiatry*, 153(3), 321–330.

Hartman, M., *et al.* (2003). Wisconsin Card Sorting Test performance in schizophrenia: the role of working memory. *Schizophrenia Research*, 63(3), 201–217.

Heaton, R.K., *et al.* (2001). Stability and course of neuropsychological deficits in schizophrenia. *Archives of General Psychiatry*, 58(1), 24–32.

Howell, D.C. (1997). *Statistical Methods for Psychology* (4th ed.). London: Wadsworth Publishing Company.

Hyman, S.E., & Fenton, W.S. (2003). Medicine. What are the right targets for psycho-pharmacology? *Science*, 299(5605), 350–351.

Ishizuka, T., *et al.* (2003). Modafinil increases histamine release in the anterior hypothalamus of rats. *Neuroscience Letters*, 339(2), 143–146.

Jasinski, D.R. (2000). An evaluation of the abuse potential of modafinil using methylphenidate as a reference. *Journal of Psychopharmacology*, 14(1), 53–60.

Koren, D., *et al.* (1998). Factor structure of the Wisconsin Card Sorting Test: dimensions of deficit in schizophrenia. *Neuropsychology*, 12(2), 289–302.

Levy, D.L., *et al.* (1993). Methylphenidate increases thought disorder in recent onset schizophrenics, but not in normal controls. *Biological Psychiatry*, 34(8), 507–514.

Lin, J.S., *et al.* (1992). Role of catecholamines in the modafinil and amphetamine induced wakefulness, a comparative pharmacological study in the cat. *Brain Research*, 591(2), 319–326.

Lin, J.S., et al. (1996). Potential brain neuronal targets for amphetamine-, methylphenidate-, and modafinil-induced wakefulness, evidenced by c-fos immunocytochemistry in the cat. *Proceedings of National Academy of Sciences of the United States of America*, 93(24), 14128–14133.

Luborsky, L. (1962). Clinician's judgments of mental health. *Archives of General Psychiatry*, 7, 407–417.

Makela, E.H., et al. (2003). Three case reports of modafinil use in treating sedation induced by antipsychotic medications. *Journal of Clinical Psychiatry*, 64(4), 485–486.

Meltzer, H.Y. (2003). Beyond control of acute exacerbation: enhancing affective and cognitive outcomes. *CNS Spectrums*, 8 (11 Suppl. 2), 16–18, 22.

Muller, U., et al. (2004). Effects of modafinil on working memory processes in humans. *Psychopharmacology (Berl)*, 177(1–2), 161–169.

Narendran, R., et al. (2002). Is psychosis exacerbated by modafinil? *Archives of General Psychiatry*, 59(3), 292–293.

Nelson, H. (1982). *National Adult Reading Test Manual*. UK: Windsor NFER-Nelson.

Pantelis, C., & Brewer, W. (1995). Neuropsychological and olfactory dysfunction in schizophrenia: relationship of frontal syndromes to syndromes of schizophrenia. *Schizophrenia Research*, 17(1), 35–45.

Pantelis, C., et al. (1999). Comparison of set-shifting ability in patients with chronic schizophrenia and frontal lobe damage. *Schizophrenia Research*, 37(3), 251–270.

Provigil. (1997). *Modafinil Datasheet*. Date of first authorisation 14 October 1997.

Randall, D.C., et al. (2004). The cognitive-enhancing properties of modafinil are limited in non-sleep-deprived middle-aged volunteers. *Pharmacology Biochemistry and Behavior*, 77(3), 547–555.

Scammell, T.E., et al. (2000). Hypothalamic arousal regions are activated during modafinil-induced wakefulness. *Journal of Neuroscience*, 20(22), 8620–8628.

Sevy, S., et al. (2005). Double-blind, placebo-controlled study of modafinil for fatigue and cognition in schizophrenia patients treated with psychotropic medications. *Journal of Clinical Psychiatry*, 66(7), 839–843.

Shelton, J., et al. (1995). Comparative effects of modafinil and amphetamine on daytime sleepiness and cataplexy of narcoleptic dogs. *Sleep*, 18(10), 817–826.

Simon, P., et al. (1994). The stimulant effect of modafinil on wakefulness is not associated with an increase in anxiety in mice. A comparison with dexamphetamine. *Psychopharmacology (Berl)*, 114(4), 597–600.

Spaulding, W.D., et al. (1999). Cognitive functioning in schizophrenia: implications for psychiatric rehabilitation. *Schizophrenia Bulletin*, 25(2), 275–289.

Spence, S.A., et al. (2005). Modafinil modulates anterior cingulate function in chronic schizophrenia. *British Journal of Psychiatry*, 187, 55–61.

Szeszko, P.R., et al. (1999). Longitudinal assessment of methylphenidate effects on oral word production and symptoms in first-episode schizophrenia at acute and stabilized phases. *Biological Psychiatry*, 45(6), 680–686.

Tanganelli, S., et al. (1994). 6-hydroxy-dopamine treatment counteracts the reduction of cortical GABA release produced by the vigilance promoting drug modafinil in the awake freely moving guinea-pig. *Neuroscience Letters*, 171(1–2), 201–204.

Tanganelli, S., et al. (1995). Modafinil and cortical gamma-aminobutyric acid outflow. Modulation by 5-hydroxytryptamine neurotoxins. *European Journal of Pharmacology*, 273(1–2), 63–71.

Taylor, F.B., & Russo, J. (2000). Efficacy of modafinil compared to dextroamphetamine for the treatment of attention deficit hyperactivity disorder in adults. *Journal of Child Adolescent Psychopharmacology*, 10(4), 311–320.

Turner, D.C., et al. (2003a). Relative lack of cognitive effects of methylphenidate in elderly male volunteers. *Psychopharmacology (Berl)*, 168(4), 455–464.

Turner, D.C., et al. (2003b). Cognitive enhancing effects of modafinil in healthy volunteers. *Psychopharmacology (Berl)*, 165(3), 260–269.

Turner, D.C., et al. (2004a). Modafinil improves cognition and response inhibition in adult attention-deficit/hyperactivity disorder. *Biological Psychiatry*, 55(10), 1031–1040.

Turner, D.C., et al. (2004b). Modafinil improves cognition and attentional set shifting in patients with chronic schizophrenia. *Neuropsychopharmacology*, 29(7), 1363–1373.

Wisor, J.P., & Eriksson, K.S. (2005). Dopaminergic–adrenergic interactions in the wake promoting mechanism of modafinil. *Neuroscience*, 132(4), 1027–1034.

Wisor, J.P., et al. (2001). Dopaminergic role in stimulant-induced wakefulness. *Journal of Neuroscience*, 21(5), 1787–1794.

Wykes, T., et al. (1999). The effects of neurocognitive remediation on executive processing in patients with schizophrenia. *Schizophrenia Bulletin*, 25(2), 291–307.

Wykes, T., et al. (2000). The prevalence and stability of an executive processing deficit, response inhibition, in people with chronic schizophrenia. *Schizophrenia Research*, 46(2–3), 241–253.

Wykes, T., et al. (2003). Are the effects of cognitive remediation therapy (CRT) durable? Results from an exploratory trial in schizophrenia. *Schizophrenia Research*, 61(2–3), 163–174.

Yu, B.P., et al. (2002). Modafinil for treatment of the negative symptoms of schizophrenia and antipsychotic-induced sedation. *Sleep*, 25 (Abstract supplement), A503–A504.

Progress in Neurotherapeutics and Neuropsychopharmacology, 1:1, 149–163 © 2006 Cambridge University Press
DOI: 10.1017/S1748232105000145   Printed in the United Kingdom

Efficacy and Tolerability of Ziprasidone and Olanzapine in Acutely Ill Inpatients with Schizophrenia or Schizoaffective Disorder: Results of a Double-Blind, Six-Week Study, with a Six-Month, Double-Blind Continuation Phase

George M. Simpson

Department of Psychiatry and the Behavioral Sciences, LAC + USC Medical Center, Psychiatric Outpatient Clinic, Los Angeles, CA, USA; Email:gsimpson@hsc.usc.edu

Antony Loebel, Lewis Warrington and Ruoyong Yang

Pfizer Inc, NY, USA

Key words: Olanzapine; zisprasidone; schizophrenia; schizoaffective disorders; clinical trial; neurotherapeutics.

Introduction and Overview

Randomized, double-blind, head-to-head trials comparing the efficacy and safety of two atypical antipsychotics continue to be relatively uncommon, though they provide data which are the most readily generalizable to decision-making in clinical practice. Approximately 20 head-to-head trials have been published to date, with the majority reporting comparisons among three atypical drugs: clozapine, risperidone, and olanzapine (Cochrane group, 2005; Tuunainen *et al.*, 2002). Few published comparator studies report data beyond 8 weeks of treatment. The results of available head-to-head trials have generally found minimal between-drug differences in efficacy. Instead, salient differences have been identified primarily in tolerability and safety outcomes.

The chronicity of schizophrenia and schizoaffective disorder, and the need for long-term therapy, make the safety and tolerability of antipsychotic drugs a central concern, both in terms of impact on compliance, and impact on longitudinal health outcomes. This is especially true since schizophrenia is associated with a 2–3-fold

Correspondence should be addressed to: George M. Simpson, MD, Department of Psychiatry and the Behavioral Sciences, LAC + USC Medical Center, IRD RM 204, Psychiatric Outpatient Clinic, 2020 Zonal Avenue, Los Angeles, CA 90033, USA, Ph: +323 226 5719; Email: gsimpson@hsc.usc.edu.

increase in all-cause mortality risk, with much of the 20% overall reduction in average life expectancy contributed by increased risk of cardiovascular (CV) and cerebrovascular mortality (Joukamaa *et al.*, 2001; Harris & Barraclough, 1998). Schizophrenic patients appear to be a metabolically vulnerable population, with a significantly higher prevalence of CV risk factors such as obesity, diabetes, and dyslipidemia (Casey *et al.*, 2004; Ryan *et al.*, 2003; Davidson *et al.*, 2001).

Emergent data suggest that atypical antipsychotics may negatively affect CV risk, though the effect may vary greatly among individual atypical drugs (Newcomer, in press; Sorensen *et al.*, 2004; Marder *et al.*, 2003). A joint American Diabetes Association/American Psychiatric Association (ADA/APA) consensus statement now recommends regular monitoring of body mass index (BMI), glucose, insulin, and lipids during treatment of schizophrenia and schizoaffective disorder with atypical antipsychotics (American Diabetes Association, American Psychiatric Association; American Association of Clinical Endocrinologists, North American Association for the Study of Obesity, 2004; Marder *et al.*, 2004). Few head-to-head trials, though, have been reported which examine in detail the comparative effect of two atypical antipsychotics drugs on metabolic parameters.

Purpose of Trial

The current study was designed to compare the safety and efficacy of ziprasidone and olanzapine in recently hospitalized patients with a primary diagnosis of schizophrenia or schizoaffective disorder. Unique features of the current trial consisted of its detailed evaluation of the effect of each drug on metabolic parameters, and the availability of 6-month double-blind continuation data in a subgroup of patients. The primary reports of the results of both the acute and continuation phases have previously been published (Simpson *et al.*, 2005, 2004).

Clinical Trial

Subjects

Male and female patients aged 18–55 years were included if they had a primary Diagnostic and Statistical Manual of Mental Disorders, Fourth Edition (DSM-IV) diagnosis of schizophrenia or schizoaffective disorder and had been hospitalized for ≤2 consecutive weeks prior to screening. To be eligible for enrollment, patients were required, at both the screen and baseline assessments, to have a Clinical Global Impression, Severity (CGI-S) score ≥4, and a Positive and Negative Syndrome Scale (PANSS) score ≥4 on at least one of the following positive symptom items: delusions, conceptual disorganization, or hallucinatory behavior. Patients were excluded for any of the following: (1) clinically significant abnormal laboratory tests, urine drug screen, or electrocardiogram (ECG); (2) history in the past year of non-response to adequate trials of two neuroleptics; (3) >14 days of olanzapine treatment (lifetime), or use of olanzapine for <14 days if the drug was discontinued due to lack of efficacy and/or poor tolerability (>10 mg dose); and (4) significant risk of suicidal or violent behavior. The protocol was approved by the Ethics Committee at each site, and study conduct was consistent with the Declaration of Helsinki. Written informed consent was obtained from all patients.

Methods

Following a 1–3 day lead-in period, patients were randomized (in a 1 : 1 ratio) to 6 weeks of double-blind treatment with either ziprasidone or olanzapine. The dose titration schedule and patient disposition during the course of the study are summarized in Figure 1. Lorazepam was permitted for control of agitation or insomnia, and benztropine was permitted for control of extrapyramidal symptoms.

At the completion of 6 weeks of double-blind treatment, patients were permitted to enroll in a 6-month continuation phase if they were outpatients, and if their CGI-Improvement score was ≤2 (much/very-much improved) or if their week 6 PANSS total score showed ≥20% reduction from baseline. Study treatment during the continuation phase consisted of flexible dosing with ziprasidone (40–80 mg BID) or olanzapine (5–15 mg/day), based on investigator clinical judgment.

Measures and Outcomes

The primary efficacy measures were the Brief Psychiatric Rating Scale (BPRS) and the CGI-S. Secondary efficacy measures included the PANSS total score and positive and negative subscales, and the Calgary Depression Scale for Schizophrenia (CDSS). Key safety measures included assessment of vital signs, body weight and BMI, physical examination, clinical laboratory tests and ECGs, the Extrapyramidal Symptoms Rating Scale (ESRS), Barnes Akathisia Scale (BAS), and Abnormal Involuntary Movement Scale (AIMS).

Analysis

The 6-week acute study was designed as a non-inferiority test of the therapeutic equivalence of ziprasidone and olanzapine on the BPRS and CGI-S scales. Equivalence on the BPRS total score was demonstrated if the two-sided 95%-confidence interval (CI) of the least squares mean difference in endpoint change scores included zero and remained within the *a priori* specified margin of 3.5 points.

Inferential analyses of change from baseline in the primary and secondary efficacy measures were based on the intent-to-treat population (ITT), last-observation-carried forward (LOCF), and tested using analysis of covariance (ANCOVA) (all

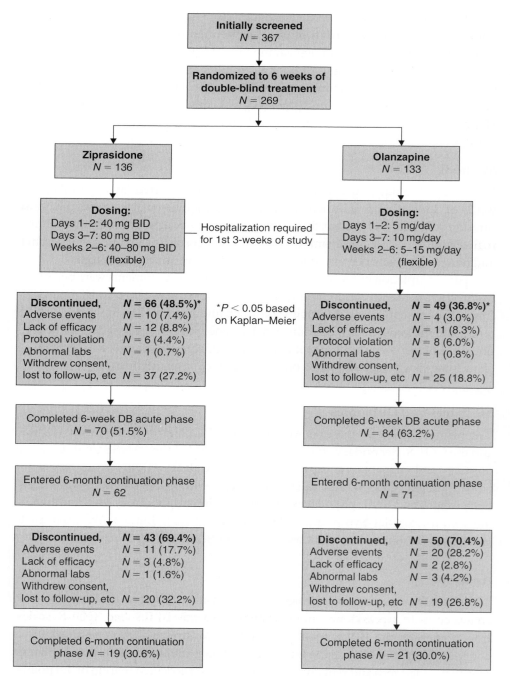

Fig. 1.
Flow diagram.

tests were two-sided; significance, 0.05). Categorical outcomes were analyzed using the Cochran–Mantel–Haenszel method (with ridit scoring).

Results

The intent-to-treat sample consisted of 269 patients who were randomized to double-blind treatment, received at least one dose of study medication, and had a baseline and post-baseline evaluation. The disposition of patients during the course of the study is summarized in Figure 1. Baseline demographic and clinical character-istics of both treatment groups were similar (Table 1), though patients on ziprasidone were somewhat less likely to be male (62% versus 69%), and had somewhat higher chronicity (median time from first psychiatric episode, 15.0 versus 12.0 years).

Efficacy

BPRS AND CGI-S

The improvement in the BPRS total score at the primary, 6-week endpoint was equivalent for ziprasidone and olanzapine (95%-CI of Δ-endpoint change: -2.36 to $+3.18$; $p = 0.77$; Figure 2(a)). Improvement in CGI-S was similarly equivalent at endpoint (95%-CI of Δ-endpoint change: -0.27 to $+0.29$; $p = 0.95$; Figure 2(b)). Improvement on both primary outcome measures was significantly greater at week 1 on ziprasidone compared to olanzapine. A Kaplan–Meier time-to-response analysis, using a 10-point improvement in BPRS total score as the criterion for clin-ical response, found a somewhat earlier median onset of treatment response on ziprasidone (15 days) compared to olanzapine (21 days; Wilcoxon p-value $= 0.092$). This earlier onset of improvement did not translate in earlier time to hospital dis-charge, which was comparable for both ziprasidone and olanzapine.

PANSS

Treatment with both drugs was associated with comparable levels of improve-ment in the PANSS total score (95%-CI of Δ-endpoint change: -4.44 to $+5.21$; $p = 0.88$; Figure 3). Similar results were observed for the PANSS positive and negative symptom scores. Consistent with BPRS and CGI-S results, onset of improvement was somewhat earlier with ziprasidone.

EFFECT ON DEPRESSIVE SYMPTOMS

Treatment with ziprasidone and olanzapine, respectively, resulted in comparable levels of endpoint improvement in the Calgary Depression Scale for Schizophrenia (-2.4 ± 0.3 versus -2.8 ± 0.3). Endpoint improvement was also comparable on the BPRS anxiety–depression factor (-2.3 ± 0.3 versus -2.4 ± 0.3). For the sub-group of patients ($n = 64$) with high depressive symptomatology at baseline (BPRS-depressed mood item score $\geqslant 4$ and anxiety–depression factor score $\geqslant 12$) there was a trend for greater endpoint improvement on ziprasidone relative to olanzapine

Table 1. **Clinical and Demographic Characteristics of Patient Sample: Baseline Data for Acute and Continuation Phases**

ACUTE PHASE BASELINE FOR TOTAL RANDOMIZED SAMPLE		
	ZIPRASIDONE (N = 136)	OLANZAPINE (N = 133)
Male (%)	61.8	69.2
Age, years (mean + SD)	37.7 ± 9.7	37.6 ± 9.7
Race (%)		
White	48.5	56.4
Black	30.9	33.8
Hispanic	15.4	5.3
Others	5.1	4.5
Schizophrenia (%)	61.8	64.7
Duration since first diagnosis, years, mean	14.6	13.3
Schizoaffective disorder (%)	38.2	35.3
Duration since first diagnosis, years, mean ± SD	16.5	14.9
Age at first psychotic episode, years, mean	22.2 ± 7.0	23.7 ± 8.1
BPRS, mean ± SD		
Total score	51.5 ± 9.5	50.7 ± 9.3
Core	15.7 ± 3.6	15.9 ± 3.3
Anxiety–depression	11.5 ± 3.6	10.8 ± 3.6
PANSS, mean ± SD		
Total score	90.0 ± 16.6	89.0 ± 16.9
Negative symptom score	22.2 ± 6.1	22.3 ± 67.2
Positive symptom score	23.2 ± 4.9	23.5 ± 5.2
CGI-S score, mean ± SD	4.9 ± 0.8	4.9 ± 0.8
CDSS total score, mean ± SD	6.0 ± 4.4	5.7 ± 4.9

ACUTE PHASE BASELINE FOR SUBGROUP ENTERING CONTINUATION PHASE		
	ZIPRASIDONE (N = 62)	OLANZAPINE (N = 71)
Male (%)	59.7	76.1
Age, years (mean ± SD)	38.0 ± 9.9	36.1 ± 9.9
Schizophrenia (%)	69.4	62.0
Duration since first diagnosis, years, mean	14.3	12.2
Schizoaffective disorder (%)	30.6	38.0
Duration since first diagnosis, years, mean	20.6	13.4
Age at first psychotic episode, years, mean ± SD	21.6 ± 7.3	23.4 ± 8.0
BPRS Total score, mean ± SD	54.5 ± 13.0	52.1 ± 10.8
PANSS, mean ± SD	93.0 ± 19.9	92.0 ± 17.9
CGI-S score, mean ± SD	5.0 ± 0.8	4.9 ± 0.7
CDSS total score, mean ± SD	6.2 ± 4.4	6.3 ± 5.6

on both the BPRS total score (-17.3 ± 1.8 versus -16.3 ± 1.8) and on the BPRS anxiety–depression factor (-5.8 ± 0.6 versus -4.4 ± 0.6; $p < 0.05$).

EFFICACY IN AFRICAN-AMERICAN SUBGROUP

For the subgroup of African-Americans ($N = 81$) improvement in the BPRS total score at LOCF-endpoint was equivalent for ziprasidone and olanzapine. The 95%-CIs of the endpoint change scores overlapped zero on the BRPS, indicating

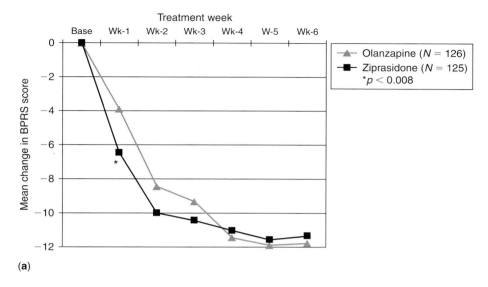

(a)

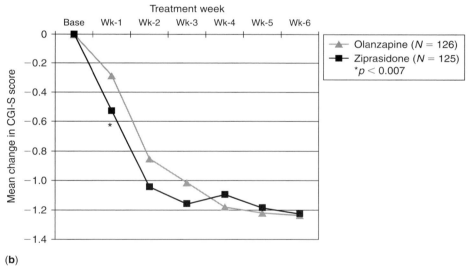

(b)

Fig. 2.
Effect of ziprasidone and olanzapine on the (**a**) BPRS total score (**b**) CGI-S score: Least square mean change scores.

that there was no significant between-group difference (95%-CI of Δ-endpoint change: −8.87 to +4.42; $p = 0.50$). Change in CGI-S was also equivalent at endpoint (95%-CI of Δ-endpoint change: −0.75 to +0.51; $p = 0.71$). Consistent with results for the total sample, improvement in BPRS total score was significantly greater at week 1 for ziprasidone compared to olanzapine (−7.8 ± 1.4 versus −3.8 ± 1.3; $p < 0.05$).

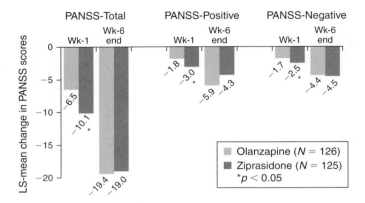

Fig. 3.
Effect of ziprasidone and olanzapine on PANSS total and factor scores: Least square mean change scores.

TOLERABILITY

The mean daily dose of study drug during the last 2 weeks of acute phase treatment was 139.0 ± 24.7 mg of ziprasidone and 13.0 ± 3.1 mg of olanzapine. 48.5% of patients on ziprasidone and 36.8% of patients on olanzapine discontinued study treatment prematurely ($p < 0.05$ on Kaplan–Meier analysis; Figure 1). Discontinuation due to adverse events was low on both ziprasidone (7.4%) and olanzapine (3.0%).

Both drugs were well-tolerated, with only a small number of adverse events occurring with an incidence of 10% or greater (Table 2). The great majority of adverse events were mild-to-moderate in severity.

There were no significant differences between ziprasidone and olanzapine on any movement disorder measures (Table 3). There was a modest tendency for patients to reduce their concomitant use of benztropine and lorazepam during the acute phase of study treatment.

When patients were asked to rate their overall preference for their current study drug compared to prior medication they had taken, the majority rated ziprasidone and olanzapine, respectively, as being slightly-to-much better on both an LOCF-endpoint analysis (63% and 61%) and a completer analysis (81% versus 70%).

SAFETY

The safety of study treatment was monitored using an extensive array of fasting laboratory tests which are summarized in Table 3. Testing focused on metabolic and CV risk parameters since schizophrenia is known to be associated with an ~20% reduction in average life expectancy, primarily due to increased CV and cerebrovascular mortality (Joukamaa *et al.*, 2001; Harris & Barraclough, 1998).

As can be seen, even by 6 weeks significant differences were consistently observed, for ziprasidone versus olanzapine, respectively, across the majority of CV risk

Table 2. **Treatment-Emergent Adverse Events (incidence ⩾10%)**

	ACUTE PHASE (6-WEEKS)	
	ZIPRASIDONE (N = 136)	OLANZAPINE (N = 133)
Somnolence (%)	22.1	20.3
Headache (%)	14.0	13.5
Dyspepsia (%)	11.8	7.5
Nausea (%)	10.3	6.0
Extrapyramidal syndrome (%)	10.3	4.5

	CONTINUATION PHASE (6-MONTHS) DATA SHOWN: TREATMENT-EMERGENT EVENTS FROM THE ACUTE PHASE BASELINE	
	ZIPRASIDONE (N = 62)	OLANZAPINE (N = 71)
Somnolence (%)	35.5	32.4
Headache (%)	25.8	18.3
Nausea (%)	17.7	5.6
Anxiety (%)	16.1	15.5
Insomnia (%)	16.1	11.3
Dyspepsia (%)	16.1	8.5
Abdominal pain (%)	12.9	5.6
Extrapyramidal syndrome (%)	12.9	4.2
Tremor (%)	11.3	5.6
Dizziness (%)	9.7	12.7
Dry mouth (%)	9.7	12.7
Pain (%)	8.1	12.7
Schizophrenic reaction (%)	4.8	15.5

parameters, including weight (+0.8 versus +3.4 kg), total cholesterol (−1.0 versus +19.5 mg/dl), LDL (−1.0 versus +13.0 mg/dl), triglycerides (−2.0 versus +26.0 mg/dl), and apolipoprotein B (−3.0 versus +9.0). In contrast, differences in QTc were not clinically or statistically significantly different (+6.08 versus +0.52 ms; Table 3).

For the total sample, Framingham risk algorithms (Wilson 1998; Wolf 1991) were applied to the on-drug changes observed in lipid profile and weight during the 6 weeks of acute treatment. The ANCOVA model yielded a net 10-year *reduction* in the risk of coronary heart disease in patients treated with ziprasidone (men, −11.1%; women, −8.7%), but an *increase* in patients treated with olanzapine (men, +7.7%; women, +0.7%) (Harrison 2004).

SIX-MONTH CONTINUATION PHASE: EFFICACY RESULTS
Continuation treatment with ziprasidone and olanzapine resulted in comparable levels of improvement in all key efficacy parameters at the 6-month continuation phase endpoint (Table 4). Treatment response was maintained at a similar rate on both ziprasidone (85.5% of completers; N = 47) compared to olanzapine (84.5%; N = 60). Symptom exacerbation, defined *a priori*, as ⩾20% worsening in the

Table 3. **Laboratory and Other Safety Parameters**

	ACUTEPHASE (6–WEEKS)	
	ZIPRASIDONE	OLANZAPINE
Movement Disorder Data		
Change in movement disorder scales, mean ± SD		
ESRS (parkinsonism, dystonia, dyskinesia)	−0.4	−0.4
Barnes Akathisia scale	0.0	−0.2
AIMS	−0.4	−0.4
Body Weight and Metabolic Data		
Change in weight, mean ± SD (kg)	0.8 + 0.01	3.4 ± 1.04[b]
Median change in serum lipid parameters		
Total cholesterol (mg/dl)	−1.0	+19.5[b]
LDL (mg/dl)	−1.0	+13.0[b]
Triglycerides (mg/dl)	−2.0	+26.0[a]
Median change in glucose metabolism parameters		
Serum insulin (μU/ml)	+0.25	+3.30[c]
C-peptide (μU/ml)	+0.16	+0.46[c]
HOMA-IR (log)	+0.06	+0.26[c]
Apolipoprotein B	−3.0	+9.0[b]
Homocysteine	−0.38	−1.06[a]
Uric acid	+0.10	+0.65[a]
ECG Data		
Change in QTc, mean (ms)	+6.08	+0.52

	CONTINUATION PHASE (6–MONTHS) DATA SHOWN: CHANGE FROM THE ACUTE PHASE BASELINE	
Movement Disorder Data		
Change in movement disorder scales, mean ± SD		
ESRS (parkinsonism, dystonia, dyskinesia)	−0.4 ± 0.3	−0.7 ± 0.3
Barnes Akathisia scale	−0.2 ± 0.4	−0.9 ± 0.3
AIMS	−0.1 ± 0.1	−0.1 ± 0.1
Body Weight and Metabolic Data		
Change in weight, mean (kg)	−0.8	+5.0[a]
Change in BMI, mean (kg)	−0.6	+1.3[a]
Median change in serum lipid parameters		
Total cholesterol (mg/dl)	−1.0	+13.0
LDL (mg/dl)	+9.0	+17.0
Median change in serum insulin (μU/ml)	+1.0	+2.0
ECG Data		
Change in QTc, mean ± SD (ms)	+1.1 ± 23.9	−5.3 ± 24.9

[a] $p < 0.01$; [b] $p < 0.001$; [c] $p < 0.08$.

PANSS total score and a CGI-S score ⩾3, was comparable at the 6-month continuation phase endpoint (log-rank $p = 0.62$ based on a Kaplan–Meier analysis).

EFFECT ON COGNITIVE FUNCTION

The effect of ziprasidone and olanzapine on cognitive function was evaluated using a battery of cognitive tests that included tests of learning and memory (Rey Auditory Verbal Learning Test; RAVLT), attention and vigilance (Trail-Making

Table 4. **Effect of Ziprasidone and Olanzapine on Key Efficacy Parameters: Change from Acute Phase Baseline to End of 6-month Continuation Phase**

	ZIPRASIDONE	OLANZAPINE
BPRS total score		
Baseline (acute), mean ± SD	54.0 ± 13.0	52.1 ± 10.8
Change at 6-month endpoint, mean ± se	−18.6 ± 2.1	−20.5 ± 1.8
CGI-S score		
Baseline (acute), mean ± SD	5.0 ± 0.8	4.9 ± 0.7
Change at 6-month endpoint, mean ± se	−1.9 ± 0.2	−2.0 ± 0.2
PANSS total score		
Baseline (acute), mean ± SD	93.0 ± 19.9	92.0 ± 17.9
Change at 6-month endpoint, mean ± se	−32.6 ± 3.8	−35.6 ± 3.3
Calgary Depression Scale for Schizophrenia		
Baseline (acute), mean ± SD	6.2 ± 4.4	6.3 ± 5.6
Change at 6-month endpoint, mean ± se	−2.8 ± 0.7	−3.0 ± 0.6

Test, part A), executive function (Trail-Making Test, part B; Wisconsin Card Sorting Test; WCST), visuomotor speed (Trail-Making Test, parts A and B), and verbal fluency (Letter Fluency Test; Category Fluency). At baseline, cognitive impairment was extensive, with 60–80% of patients showing significant impairment on each individual test. After 6 months of continuation treatment, cognitive function had normalized, depending on the individual test, in approximately 20–40% of patients (Figure 4). The degree of normalization of cognitive function was comparable for both ziprasidone and olanzapine, and treatment with both drugs was associated with markedly greater cognitive effects than were observed after 6 weeks of acute therapy. There was no correlation between improvement in positive or negative symptoms and improvement in cognitive function, suggesting the extent to which this may be an independent outcome domain. More detail on these results are presented in a previous report (Harvey, in press).

SIX-MONTH CONTINUATION PHASE: SAFETY RESULTS

Long-term treatment was generally well tolerated with most adverse events being in the mild-to-moderate range of severity. Discontinuation due to treatment-related adverse events was similarly low for both ziprasidone (3.2%) and olanzapine (2.8%). For olanzapine, there were significant within-group increases in median fasting insulin (+2.0 μU/ml) ($p = 0.003$), total cholesterol (+13.0 mg/dl) ($p = 0.03$), and low-density lipoprotein cholesterol (+17.0 mg/dl) ($p = 0.04$). For ziprasidone, none of the within-group changes in fasting insulin (+1.0 μU/ml) ($p = 0.14$), total cholesterol (−1.0 mg/dl) ($p = 0.98$), and low-density lipoprotein cholesterol (+9.0 mg/dl) ($p = 0.29$) were significant. Olanzapine treatment was also associated with significant increase in median values for aspartate aminotransferase (6.0 U/l) ($p < 0.001$) and alanine aminotransferase (7.0 U/l) ($p < 0.01$). Neither treatment significantly affected vital signs. Across both phases of study

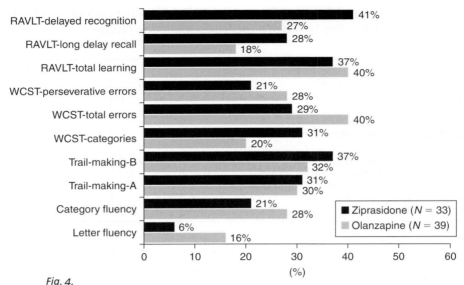

Fig. 4.

Normalization of cognitive function on ziprasidone versus olanzapine: Results at 6 months.
Source: Simpson *et al.*, 2004.

treatment there was one treatment-related serious adverse event on ziprasidone
(diabetes mellitus), and one on olanzapine (acute change in mental status).

Discussion

The results of the current study demonstrate that ziprasidone and olanzapine have
comparable efficacy, both acutely and after 6 months, across all key measures of
psychosis, depressive symptoms, and global illness severity.

Several efficacy findings are notable. First, a Kaplan–Meier analysis found a
trend-significant earlier time-to-response on ziprasidone (15 days) compared to
olanzapine (21 days). Earlier onset did not result in earlier discharge from the hospital, though investigators were discouraged from discharging patients early in the
current study. This difference in time-to-response needs to be confirmed by additional double-blind, comparator trials which are also designed to evaluate
whether this clinical finding has any pharmacoeconomic impact.

Secondly, continuation treatment for up to 6 months resulted in sustained
improvement, with no relapse, in 85.5% of patients on ziprasidone and 84.5% of
patients on olanzapine. Inferences about long-term efficacy of ziprasidone and olanzapine are severely limited by the high attrition rate observed in the 6-month continuation phase of the trial. This is a problem endemic to most long-term schizophrenia
treatment studies. Time-to-attrition was significantly earlier on ziprasidone compared to olanzapine. This may be attributable, in part, to use of a relatively low starting dose of 80 mg/day. Both clinical experience (Weiden, 2002) and clinical trials

data (Joyce, 2004) suggest that initiating ziprasidone therapy at higher doses (120–160 mg/day) may reduce the incidence of activation symptomatology, and make patients significantly less likely to discontinue treatment within the first 6 months than when therapy is initiated at a dose of 80 mg/day or lower. Interestingly, the attrition rate in controlled clinical trials tends to be higher than in actual clinical practice. For example, a recent analysis of a medical and pharmacy claims database found average duration of therapy to be higher on both ziprasidone (228 days) and olanzapine (201 days) than we found in this study (Harrison, 2005). The higher attrition in clinical trials may be due either to study fatigue (from the burden of numerous ratings, laboratory tests and other evaluations) or to differences in the study sample.

A third efficacy finding was the benefit of both drugs in improving symptoms of psychosis in a subgroup of African-American patients. The magnitude of benefit appeared to be similar across races. Onset of treatment response also was earlier in this subgroup. More research is needed which examines the efficacy and safety of individual drugs on various ethnic populations.

A final efficacy finding of note was the beneficial effect of both ziprasidone and olanzapine on cognitive function. More than two-thirds of patients had abnormal cognitive function at pre-treatment baseline. By the end of 6 months of continuation therapy, cognitive function had normalized in the majority of patients. Improvement was not clearly correlated with remission of either positive or negative symptoms, emphasizing the extent to which cognitive function is an independent outcome domain.

In contrast to the modest between-drug differences in efficacy, ziprasidone and olanzapine were found to have significant differences in safety parameters, especially those relating to weight and metabolic parameters. Six weeks of treatment with ziprasidone resulted in minimal effects on weight, and minimal changes in blood lipids or measures of glycemic control. In contrast, acute treatment with olanzapine was associated with significant increases in weight, fasting lipids, fasting insulin, and homeostatic model assessment (HOMA-IR (log)), a well-established measure of insulin resistance. The increases on olanzapine in weight, glucose metabolism, and lipids were sustained during long-term treatment.

The differential effect of ziprasidone and olanzapine on weight and metabolic parameters has significant potential impact on health outcomes, as illustrated by the pilot analysis using Framingham risk algorithms. The net *difference* in CV risk contributed by use of olanzapine relative to ziprasidone is approximately 10% in men and 20% in women. The differentially higher CV risk associated with olanzapine must be included in benefit-risk estimates that inform clinical decision-making, especially where maintenance therapy is being considered.

In conclusion, the results of this two-phase study found both ziprasidone and olanzapine to be comparable across all efficacy outcomes, with the possible exception of an earlier time-to-onset of treatment effect, favoring ziprasidone, which requires confirmation by additional head-to-head clinical trials. In contrast, ziprasidone appears to have a notably more favorable cardiovascular profile, which may favor its use in clinical circumstances where maintenance therapy is an important consideration.

Acknowledgment

This study was supported by Pfizer Inc.

References

American Diabetes Association; American Psychiatric Association; American Association of Clinical Endocrinologists; North American Association for the Study of Obesity. (2004). Consensus development conference on antipsychotic drugs and obesity and diabetes. *Diabetes Care*, 27, 596–601.

Casey, D.E., Haupt, D.W., Newcomer, J.W., Henderson, D.C., Sernyak, M.J., Davidson, M., Lindenmayer, J.P., Manoukian, S.V., Banerji, M.A., Lebovitz, H.E., & Hennekens, C.H. (2004). Antipsychotic-induced weight gain and metabolic abnormalities: Implications for increased mortality in patients with schizophrenia. *Journal of Clinical Psychiatry*, 65 (Suppl. 7), 4–18.

Cochrane Group. (2005). Risperidone versus olanzapine for schizophrenia. *Cochrane Database System Review*, April 18; (2): CD005237.

Davidson, S., Judd, F., Jolley, D., Hocking, B., Thompson, S., & Hyland, B. (2001). Cardiovascular risk factors for people with mental illness. *Australian and New Zealand Journal of Psychiatry*, 35, 196–202.

Harris, E.C., & Barraclough, B. (1998). Excess mortality of mental disorder. *British Journal of Psychiatry*, 173, 11–53.

Harrison, D.J., Leaderer, M.C., Loebel, A., & Murray, S. (2004). Ziprasidone vs. olanzapine: change in CHD risk during a 6-week trial. Poster presentation, *157th Annual Meeting of the American Psychiatric Association*, New York, May.

Harrison, D.J., Joyce, A.T., & Ollendorf, D.A. (2005). Impact of Atypical Agents on Outcomes of Care in Schizophrenia. Poster presentation, *158th Annual Meeting of the American Psychiatric Association*, Atlanta, May.

Harvey, P.D., Bowie, C.R., & Loebel, A. (in press). Neuropsychological normalization with long-term atypical antipsychotic treatment: results of a 6-month, randomized, double-blind comparison of ziprasidone vs. Olanzapine.

Joukamaa, M., Heliovaara, M., Knekt, P., Aromaa, A., Raitasalo, R., & Lehtinen, V. (2001). Mental disorders and cause-specific mortality. *British Journal of Psychiatry*, 179, 498–502.

Joyce, A.T., Harrison, D.J., & Ollendorf, D.A. (2004). Effect of ziprasidone initial dosing on discontinuation. Poster presentation, *157th Annual Meeting of the American Psychiatric Association*, New York, May.

Marder, S.R., McQuade, R.D., Stock, E., Kaplita, S., Marcus, R., Safferman, A.Z., Saha, A., Ali, M., & Iwamoto, T. (2003). Aripiprazole in the treatment of schizophrenia: safety and tolerability in short-term, placebo-controlled trials. *Schizophrenia Research*, 61, 123–136.

Marder, S.R., Essock, S.M., Miller, A.L., Buchanan, R.W., Casey, D.E., Davis, J.M., Kane, J.M., Lieberman, J.A., Schooler, N.R., Covell, N., Stroup, S., Weissman, E.M.,

Wirshing, D.A., Hall, C.S., Pogach, L., Pi-Sunyer, X., Bigger, J.T. Jr., Friedman, A., Kleinberg, D., Yevich, S.J., Davis, B., & Shon, S. (2004). Physical health monitoring of patients with schizophrenia. *American Journal of Psychiatry*, 161, 1334–1349.

Newcomer, J.W. (2005). Atypical antipsychotics and metabolic effects: a comprehensive literature review. *CNS Drugs*, 19 (suppl 1): 1–93.

Ryan, M.C., Collins, P., & Thakore, J.H. (2003). Impaired fasting glucose tolerance in first-episode, drug-naive patients with schizophrenia. *American Journal of Psychiatry*, 160, 284–289.

Simpson, G.M., Glick, I.D., Weiden, P.J., Romano, S.J., & Siu, C.O. (2004). Randomized, controlled, double-blind multicenter comparison of the efficacy and tolerability of ziprasidone and olanzapine in acutely ill inpatients with schizophrenia or schizoaffective disorder. *American Journal of Psychiatry*, 161, 1837–1847.

Simpson, G.M., Weiden, P., Pigott, T., Murray, S., Siu, C.O., & Romano, S.J. (2005). Six-month, blinded, multicenter continuation study of ziprasidone versus olanzapine in schizophrenia. *American Journal of Psychiatry*, 162, 1535–1538.

Sorensen, S.V., Leaderer, M.C., Harrison, D.J., Prasad, M., Hollenbeak, C., Dugar, A., & Remak, E. (2004). Psychiatric and metabolic outcomes of antipsychotics in schizophrenia. Poster presentation, *157th Annual Meeting of the American Psychiatric Association*, New York, May.

Tuunainen, A., Wahlbeck, K., & Gilbody, S. (2002). Newer atypical antipsychotic medication in comparison to clozapine: a systematic review of randomized trials. *Schizophrenia Research*, 56, 1–10.

Weiden, P.J., Iqbal, N., Mendelowitz, A.J., Tandon, R., Zimbroff, D.L., & Ross, R. (2002). Best clinical practice with ziprasidone: update after one year of experience. *Journal of Psychiatric Practice*, 8, 81–97.

Wilson, P.W., D'Agostino, R.B., Levy, D., Belanger, A.M., Silbershatz, H., & Kannel, W.B. (1998). Prediction of coronary heart disease using risk factor categories. *Circulation*, 97, 1837–1847.

Wolf, P.A., Abbott, R.D., & Kannel, W.B. (1991). Atrial fibrillation as an independent risk factor for stroke: the Framingham Study. *Stroke*, 22, 983–988.

Progress in Neurotherapeutics and Neuropsychopharmacology, 1:1, 165–167 © 2006 Cambridge University Press
DOI: 10.1017/S1748232105000157   Printed in the United Kingdom

Subject Index

Progress in Neurotherapeutics and Neuropsychopharmacology, 1:1, 169 © 2006 Cambridge University Press
DOI: 10.1017/S1748232105000169   Printed in the United Kingdom

Author Index